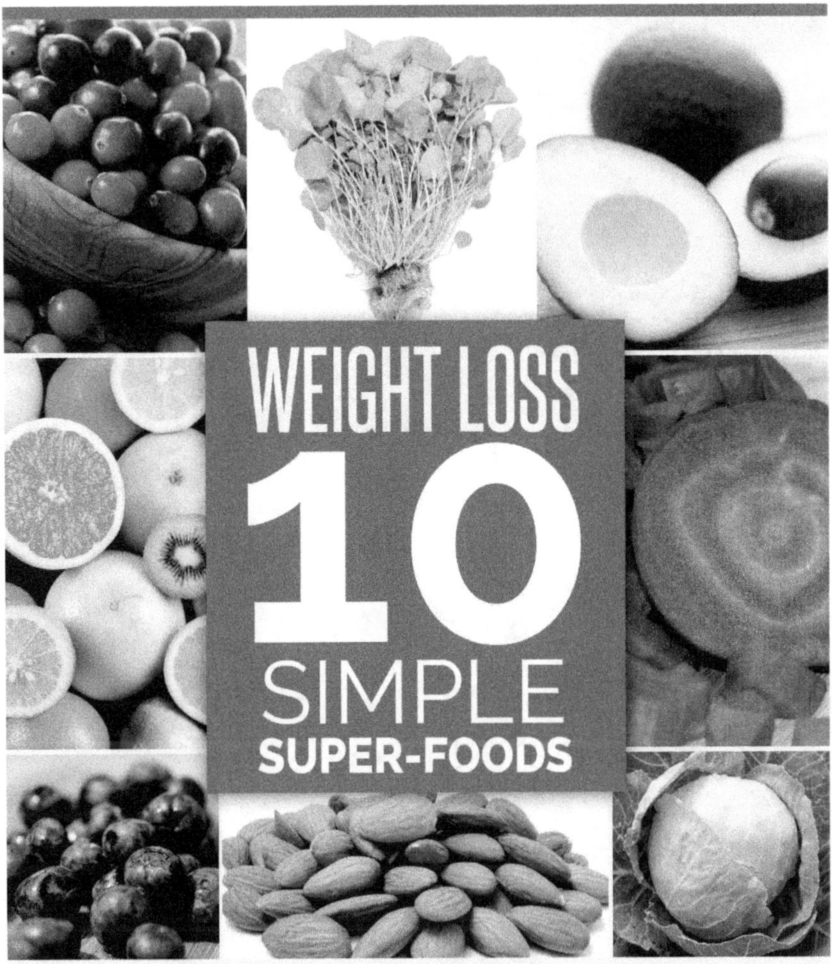

WEIGHT LOSS

10

SIMPLE
SUPER-FOODS

That will help you **Lose weight naturally,**
produce More **Energy natually**, and
feel great everyday!

DR. A. THOMAS SPENCER

CONTENTS...

Part 2: Keeping the Weight off

Weight Loss 10 Commandments

Drink Water	• 8-10 cups a day
Eat Protein with every Meal	• Healthy protein intake gives improved energy.
Always Eat Breakfast	• Start your day off right.
Eat Before and After you Excersise	• You need Fuel!
Eat what grows on the Trees	• Eat whats green!
Don't Drink Calories	• Don't drink the Liquid Candy Bars!
Eat Salad Everyday	• Can I say, Regulation!
Eat 6 Small Meals a Day	• Metabolism on Fire!
Eat Unprocessed Foods	• Processed is not HEALTY!
Do Your Very Best	• You can Acheive if you Beleive!

WEIGHT LOSS FACTS & MYTHS & TIPS

- *1 pound is the equivalent of 3500 calories*

- *Just because it says "Fat-Free" on the label, it is not always good.*

- *Sugar is the number one killer in the world*

- *Supplements can never replace nutrition from real food*

- *Its not a diet that will work, but a lifestyle change*

- *Don't Always believe the Scale*

- *Snacking Is Always a Bad Idea (Not true. Your weight is based on your calorie intake. If you take in too many calories, than you put on weight and vice versa.)*

- *Carbohydrates are actually an important source of energy*

- *Skipping meals can lead to weight gain*

- *Your genes determine your metabolism and body weight (Only 25% of your genes determine body weight)*

- *Your body won't burn fat unless you exercise for more than 20 minutes. (You burn calories around the clock)*

- *Certain foods, like grapefruit, celery, or cabbage soup, can burn fat and make you lose weight. (There are no foods that burn fat)*

- *Skipping meals is a good way to lose weight. (People who do this are shown to be heavier than people who eat small meals throughout the day)*

- *Eating after 8 p.m. causes weight gain (It doesn't matter when you eat, what matters is how many calories you intake)*

- *Exercise must be strenuous and must be done at a certain intensity and for a certain amount of time to be any help in losing weight*

- *It is possible to change dietary habits to lose weight and still eat meals that are satisfying, good tasting, and nutritious*

- *One gram of fat contains more than twice the calories of one gram of carbohydrate or protein*

Introduction

What do I eat?

Nutritionists get that question all the time. Studies have shown that the average person has little understanding or a low **Nutritional IQ**. They really don't know what to eat at all! Part of the reasoning, stems from schools throughout the world not making nutrition a focus in the classroom. Because of our lack of knowledge, we are often tricked or fooled by companies in their labeling of product, and commercials promoting the nutritional benefits of their food. We see the tricks daily with slogans like "fat free, low fat, heart healthy, low sodium, low cholesterol," to make the everyday consumers feel that they are eating healthy foods. The truth is that many companies use this propaganda to get us to buy their products. And it is more cost effective for companies and restaurants to use processed food, non-organic, and simple sugars to gain an audience, following, and more importantly a profit for their business. It is time to get a better understanding and educate ourselves on nutrition. Don't short change yourself with non-nutritious foods. Which is why after this introduction, we focus immediately on the **Nutrition Label.** Understanding this label is critical in building your nutritional IQ. The label covers exactly what the contents hold. Do not always believe what the food producers put on the front of their items. This nutrition label tells the truth!

10 simple foods to have in your fridge!

Nutrition is one of the most important facets in life. The goal of this book is to break down the most important points when it comes to achieving weight loss with everyday eating. It focuses on **Ten Foods** that naturally help our bodies lose excess weight, and boost our metabolism naturally. With such a high pace society, simplification is key. Keeping these ten foods in your refrigerator will make a dramatic difference!

Selecting the Ten Foods for this book

Much time and effort was put into the selection of the top ten foods. Narrowing down to just ten items was a lengthy process. Our nutrition committee used a rating scale based on four factors.

1.*Metabolism enhancement*

2.*Detoxifying characteristics*

3.*Digestive system enhancement*

4.*Immune system boost.*

PURPOSE of this Book

The main purpose of this book is to focus on eating the best foods (that benefit your body) possible daily and keeping the weight off. You will be able to eliminate all of the toxins in your body and then replace them by feeding your body with healthier, nutritious food...essentially detoxifying your body, losing unwanted body fat, and producing more energy naturally. Your metabolism will increase dramatically, helping you lose those extra pounds. This will be a major force in defending your body against various types of diseases and restoring your body to its maximum health. You will read about ten different kinds of foods, the 'top 10 simple super foods', that will both restore and maintain that your body, and furthermore help your digestion system, enhance your metabolism, reinforce your body's immune system, and facilitate losing weight.

Plain and simple, if you want to embark on the journey ahead to improve your body and maintain the newfound levels of health you will reach, this book is a good start for you. And you don't have to embark on that journey by washing down pills or medicine, or even fancy, expensive smoothies. But by simply making a run to your local grocery store. Believe it or not, there are lots of delicious foods in the market place that are very friendly to detoxification properties. Not only are these foods delicious and generally inexpensive, but also they will enhance your energy and make your body healthier. Including just a few of these nutritious foods into your daily diet alone is a safe bet for cleansing your body of toxins and making it more healthy. There are no special diets or expensive supplements required for you to purchase. All the information you need to change your lifestyle of eating and produce a healthier person is right here in this book!

Make cleansing your body and filling it with nutritious foods both your goal and your dream. Enhance your nutritional IQ by educating yourself. Understand what foods are beneficial for your body and how they add to your health. The biggest challenge you will face is to stay consistent and not give into foods that are bad for you. To discipline yourself and scale back drastically on unhealthy foods that you're use to eating. Once you do that, then improving your body will be a walk in the park, and you will succeed where others have failed. You can do it!

You Have Lost The Weight, Now What?

As a *bonus*, we added a second part to this book, which focuses on how to keep the weight off once it is gone. Your body will plateau. Plateau is a natural phenomenon. Your body is a master at adaptation, but we can trick it! Thankfully there are many different tactics, through exercise and eating, which can be used to confuse your body and get it past this difficult stage. We give you the tools and knowledge to have long-term success!

Thanks again for downloading this book, I hope you enjoy it!

How to Understand and Use the Nutrition Facts Label

Nutrition Facts

Serving Size 1 cup (236ml)
Servings Per Container 1

Amount Per Serving

Calories 80   Calories from Fat 0

% Daily Value*

Total Fat 0g	**0%**
Saturated Fat 0g	**0%**
Trans Fat 0g	
Cholesterol Less than 5mg	**0%**
Sodium 120mg	**5%**
Total Carbohydrate 11g	**4%**
Dietary Fiber 0g	**0%**
Sugars 11g	
Protein 9g	**17%**

Vitamin A 10%	•	Vitamin C 4%
Calcium 30% •	Iron 0% •	Vitamin D 25%

*Percent Daily Values are based on a 2,000 calorie diet. Your daily values may be higher or lower depending on your calorie needs.

Most people read nutritional labels to see how many calories they will be consuming. But it is important to realize there is a great abundance of information on nutritional labels that people should be paying attention to. For example, if you are keeping track of your calorie intake it is important to check how many servings are in the item that you are eating. You would be surprised how many times there are several servings in the one item you are eating which means you are consuming more than just the calories per one serving. Another benefit is seeing the vitamins and nutrients you are getting, along with your daily percentage of the good (fiber) with the bad (saturated fats).

A Deeper Look At The Nutrition Label

The content in the top portion of the label (like in our examples below) can vary depending on the item; but it always contains serving size, calories, and nutrient information. The bottom part portion of the nutritional label will tell you what the percentage of your daily value for an item is based on. In most cases the percentage is based on a 2,000 to 2,500 calorie diet. This footnote provides recommended dietary information for important nutrients, including fats, sodium and fiber.

Serving Size

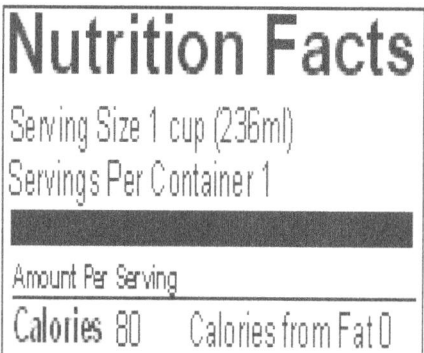

Serving Size 1 cup (236ml) Servings Per Container 1

When going over a nutrition label one of the first things you will notice is the severing size and how many per container. Serving sizes usually go by a base amount like cups for example.

The number of calories and amount of nutrients listed on the nutrition label is based on serving size. Many of times there are more than one serving for that item. So pay close attention so you know how many servings you are consuming.

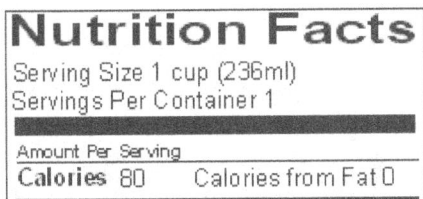

Calorie Intake

A calorie is the measurement of how much energy you get from the food you eat. Which is why it is important to consume only a certain amount of calories. If you consume too much then that left over energy turns into fat and is stored so the body can use it as needed.

Useful Guide For Calories General Guide to Calories

1. 50 Calories is low
2. 100 Calories is moderate
3. 500 Calories or more is high

The **General Guide to Calories** is based on a 2,000-calorie diet.
Eating too many calories per day is correlated to weight gain and obesity.

Nutrients that Need to be Limited

Nutrition Facts

Serving Size 1 cup (236ml)
Servings Per Container 1

Amount Per Serving

Calories 80   Calories from Fat 0

	% Daily Value*
Total Fat 0g	0%
Saturated Fat 0g	0%
Trans Fat 0g	
Cholesterol Less than 5mg	0%
Sodium 120mg	5%

Some of the main nutrients that need to be limited are fat, saturated fat, trans fat, cholesterol, and sodium. Consuming too much of these nutrients will increase your risk of heart disease, high blood pressure, and some cancers.

Maintain These Nutrients

Total Carbohydrate 11g	4%
Dietary Fiber 0g	0%
Sugars 11g	
Protein 9g	17%

Vitamin A 10% • Vitamin C 4%	
Calcium 30% • Iron 0% • Vitamin D 25%	

*Percent Daily Values are based on a 2,000 calorie diet. Your daily values may be higher or lower depending on your calorie needs.

There are nutrients on the nutrition label that most Americans don't consume enough of these nutrients being fiber, vitamin C, vitamin A, calcium, and iron. Consuming the daily amounts recommended will improve health and reduce the risk of developing some diseases and illnesses. For instance, consuming fiber helps with health waste function. Also consuming enough calcium helps reduce the risk of osteoporosis.

How Daily Values Relate to Daily Percentage

Nutrition Facts

Serving Size 1 cup (236ml)
Servings Per Container 1

Amount Per Serving

Calories 80   Calories from Fat 0

% Daily Value*

Total Fat 0g	0%
Saturated Fat 0g	0%
Trans Fat 0g	
Cholesterol Less than 5mg	0%
Sodium 120mg	5%
Total Carbohydrate 11g	4%
Dietary Fiber 0g	0%
Sugars 11g	
Protein 9g	17%

Vitamin A 10%   •   Vitamin C 4%

Calcium 30% • Iron 0% • Vitamin D 25%

*Percent Daily Values are based on a 2,000 calorie diet. Your daily values may be higher or lower depending on your calorie needs.

The recommended daily value is based on a board of doctors. It is to be used as a guide for maintaining a healthy weight. Although calorie intake can be different for every individual depending on, age, and activity level, and so on, it can still be a helpful guide.

The Percent Daily Value (%DV):

Nutrition Facts

Serving Size 1 cup (236ml)
Servings Per Container 1

Amount Per Serving

Calories 80   Calories from Fat 0

	% Daily Value*
Total Fat 0g	0%
Saturated Fat 0g	0%
Trans Fat 0g	
Cholesterol Less than 5mg	0%
Sodium 120mg	5%
Total Carbohydrate 11g	4%
Dietary Fiber 0g	0%
Sugars 11g	
Protein 9g	17%

Vitamin A 10%   •   Vitamin C 4%

Calcium 30% • Iron 0% • Vitamin D 25%

*Percent Daily Values are based on a 2,000 calorie diet. Your daily values may be higher or lower depending on your calorie needs.

The percentage for the nutrients in the food product is all calculated based on a doctor recommended 2,000-calorie diet. Most people are unaware of how many grams or milligrams they need to consume in a day to get 100% of the nutrients their bodies need. So having the percentage listed for you makes it easy to calculate how much you have consumed and how much more you may need to hit your daily percentage.

Best Ways To Use Nutrition Label

There are several benefits to using the nutritional label. One way is that it is a great aid in comparing the same product. For example, you want to get the healthiest yogurt with the lowest calories and the highest calcium possible. All you have to do is compare labels to see which one has the lowest amount of calories per serving and which one has the highest amount of calcium per serving.

You can compare percentages to make sure your daily fat consumption is limited. This is a great benefit if you are on a current diet such as a high protein and high fiber diet. Keeping track of your daily consumption will help you maintain those high levels desired. Also if your main concern is to watch your calorie intake then using the nutrition label will aid in tracking your daily intake.

Are you paying attention?

Here is a Question. What was the number circled in red on the Nutrition label?

a. 20%

b. 40%

c. 30%

d. None of the above.

Yes, that part was **boring**, but did it help? The nutrition label is all that we have to know what the contents are in the food we eat. You would be surprised at how many people pay it no attention.

NOW LETS LEARN THE TEN FOODS THAT YOU MUST EAT TO LOSE WEIGHT NATURALLY, PRODUCE MORE ENERGY AND FEEL GREAT EVERYDAY!

Almonds

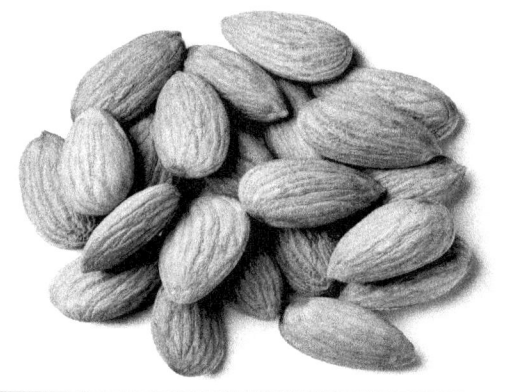

Almonds are a very nutritious snack with far more health benefits than most people realize. They are the healthiest of all tree nuts because they are packed with minerals that are very beneficial to your body. Only a small handful per day will enhance the health of your heart and lead to losing weight, in addition to fighting various types of devastating diseases such as diabetes.

Almonds are an excellent source of food to detoxify your body. They are one of the best nut sources for Vitamin E, as just one ounce of almonds carries 7.3mg of alpha-tocopherol, or 35T of the daily-recommended intake, which is the form of vitamin the human body favors. Almonds are also rich in magnesium, calcium, proteins and fiber. As a result, almonds are efficient in stabilizing blood sugar levels and removing bad substances from the body.

Something that many people don't realize is that almonds are actually the seeds of a fruit, very closely related to plums and peaches. Almond milk also serves as an alternative to cow's milk, which is not rich in detox diets. Not only that, but almond milk is also better tasting in comparison to plant alternatives. Almond milk is easily accessible at grocery and health food stores, or can be homemade.

There are also many ways to enjoy almonds. They can be taken by adding almonds or almond milk to a smoothie or you can chop up almonds and add them to vegetable or salad dishes, cereals, or in pesto as a substitute for peanut butter and pine nuts. In addition, just eating plain almonds in your hand is a tasty and nutritious snack. This way, you can make trail mix to eat while on the road or taking a hike into the beautiful mountains. All you have to do is combine a handful of almonds with some fruit, and you're good to go.

Top Ten Reasons to eat Almonds everyday

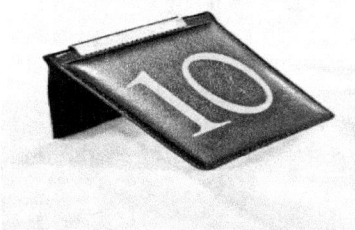

1. Lower Your Cholesterol

2. Regulate Your Blood Pressure

3. Prevent Cancer

4. They Protect Against Diabetes

5. Lose Weight with Nuts

6. Boost Your Energy

7. Reduce the Risk of Heart Disease

8. Prevent Birth Defects

9. Improve Your Brainpower

10. They Taste Wonderful!

Per day, you will need to eat about twenty-three almonds to earn the nutrients needed for your daily diet. These twenty there almonds contain one hundred and sixty calories from thirteen grams of healthy unsaturated fats and only one gram of saturated fat. Almonds are loaded with calcium, vitamin E, potassium and magnesium, but they are also a huge source of fiber and proteins. To top it all off, they are also very low in cholesterol and sugar. This makes almonds among the healthiest of foods to eat, and adding them to your diet will be a huge help in detoxifying your body. Overall, almonds are the healthiest of all nuts due to their high amounts of minerals such as protein, fiber and calcium.

Eating one or two ounces of almonds every day will be a major factor in limiting the risk of heart disease. This is due to the high levels of magnesium contained within almonds that serve to prevent heart disease by also preventing hypertension. Almonds can also prevent heart disease when it comes to cholesterol. In the body, there are essentially two types of cholesterol: 'good' cholesterol and 'bad' cholesterol. Good cholesterol is called HDL cholesterol, while bad cholesterol is called LDL cholesterol. Due to the high levels of magnesium in almonds, levels of HDL cholesterol are raised, greatly increasing health benefits and lowering the risk of heart disease. Almonds also not only contain no LDL cholesterol, but they also work to decrease existing levels of LDL cholesterol in the body.

One of the most important things to remember when trying to become healthy is to watch your weight. Maintaining a healthy weight is immensely beneficial to increasing your body's health, and almonds serve well when it comes to weight maintenance. The fiber, protein and fat contained in the almonds make you feel full and help you resist the urge to eat more food than you should be eating. In addition, the magnesium in almonds regulates the levels of blood sugar in the body, which helps immensely in reducing your urge to eat more food. But eating food aside, almonds can further more help you lose weight due to blocking your body incorporation of calories. The only thing to be careful about here is to remember that almonds themselves are high in calories, so as a result you need to remember to limit how many almonds you have to the twenty-three nuts, or one ounce, per day. As long as you don't eat too many almonds and not too few, your body's health will enhance immensely.

As stated in the opening paragraph of the chapter, almonds also serve to fight various types of devastating diseases. Almonds can uphold gastrointestinal health, and perhaps even enhance it, due to the pre-biotic properties of the almonds' fiber content, contributing to the health of the gastrointestinal tract. These are food substances that do not digest, meaning they provide for a healthy balance of good bacteria in the intestinal tract. But more importantly, almonds can also serve to be a major contributor in your body's fight against diabetes. Almonds can very effectively fight diabetes without increasing your weight, decreasing your energy for high levels of physical activity, or disturbing your daily intake of calories.

All in all, almonds are an incredibly nutritious food source that will help to detoxify your body. They are available in a very wide range of preparations, from raw, unsalted almonds to roasted almonds. But no matter which whey you prepare or prefer your almonds, they are always fully loaded with extremely high levels of nutrients, minerals and calories, so they are healthy no matter what. What's more, no matter how you prepare them, almonds are lacking in poor fats and abundant in natural beneficial fats, though often some of the beneficial fats are cooked away when almonds are roasted.

If you have decided you want to detoxify your body, then a major step forward you can take is to start including just twenty-three or one ounce of, almonds in your daily diet. If you can do that, then you will begin to see immediate health benefits and your body will already start working to cleanse itself from the inside. And while you can't completely cleanse your body by simply adding those twenty-three almonds to your diet, they are definitely a major step forward in the right direction.

Avocados

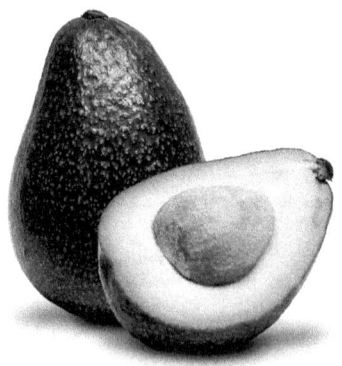

Avocados are very rich in monounsaturated fats. They burn very easy and can be used for energy.

Facts: Avocados also have twice the potassium of a banana.

Many people turn away from avocados due to the high levels of fat in its content. Indeed, during the diet craze of the 80's through the 90s, many people avoid avocados extensively. First of all, it is true that avocados contain a high level of fat. But what a lot of people don't realize is that avocados are high in monounsaturated fat, which is very healthy for the heart and doesn't interfere with the balancing of the other fatty acids in a person's diet.

10 Reasons To Eat Avocados

1. **Studies show that avocados aide in prostate cancer prevention.**
2. **Cancer Defense: (especially oral cancer)**
3. **Eye Health**
4. **Breast Cancer prevention**
5. **Heart Health**
6. **Lowers bad cholesterol**
7. **The best source for Vitamin E**
8. **Will aide in Nutrient absorption**

9. Stroke prevention
10. An excellent source of Glutathione

Truth be told, fat will actually be indispensible if you are embarking on a detoxification diet. Fats are a tremendous aid in releasing bile from the gallbladder, which in turn terminates other toxins in the body and absorbs vitamins that are fat-soluble such as vitamin A, D, E and K. After all, one of the main purposes of taking a detox diet in the first place is to get rid of all the toxins in your body, right?

Avocados also hold high levels of Vitamins B5 and E, as well as potassium. If you include one half of a cup of avocados in your daily diet, this is equal to eight grams of dietary fiber in your body. As a result of this newfound evidence, avocados are becoming extensively popular as a detox food. In addition, avocados can even serve as alternatives to multiple unhealthy foods that you will need to scale back on, if not eliminate entirely, when on your detox diet.

Avocados contain buttery textures that add creaminess to smoothies or other beverages, allowing you to eliminate unhealthy milks and creams from your diet. You can also use avocados as an extra in salsa, and as a dipping sauce or as a dressing for salads. While this definitely adds plenty of taste to salads, it's been scientifically proven that avocado dressing or dipping sauce for salads is extremely healthy for your body. It absorbs key antioxidants, such as beta-carotene and lycopene, and when added to a salad containing components such as spinach, lettuce, and carrots, this increases those absorptions to between two hundred to four hundred percent. Carotenoids in particular are soluble in fat, and the avocado would provide extra fat.

It's also been scientifically proven to show that how you prepare your avocado does make a huge difference as to how it affects your health. Most of the carotenoids in avocados are located in the dark green flesh beneath the skin. If you wedge your kitchen knife into that flesh, you eliminate many of the carotenoids that absorb the key antioxidants. Instead, a more effective way to 'peel' an avocado is by hand, and not by knife or tool. All you have to do is cut the avocado from end-to-end, and end up with two long avocado halves still connected by the seed in the middle. Then, you twist them in different directions until they pull apart.

Next, continue to cut long sections of the avocado to as many pieces as you like (four is the typical number). All you have to do then is use your fingers to peel the edge of the skin. As a result, you will have an avocado that is peeled but that also holds all of the carotenoids. This is the best way to prepare a detox avocado.

There are many other sources of carotenoids, like in tomatoes, carrots, or other bright red vegetables. However, research studies have found that avocados contain even more carotenoids than these other sources. While carrots and tomatoes are also excellent sources of carotenoids, well, avocados are an even more excellent source. This is because avocados contain a wide variety of different types of carotenoids that are key in the anti-inflammatory assets of it. Not only do avocados contain the most well known types of carotenoids, they also include many lesser-known ones that wouldn't be found in red vegetables like carrots or tomatoes.

Avocados basically contain three kinds of fat: beat-sitosterol, campesterol, and stigmasterol. These fats are all a part of the phytosterols fat, and it is because of these fats working in our inflammatory system that our inflammation is kept under control. Due to the anti-inflammatory positives of these fats, studies have revealed that avocados can also serve to help problems with arthritis.

Fatty alcohols in avocados, particularly the polyhydroxylated fatty alcohols, can also help keep inflammation under control. In addition, these fatty alcohols are most commonly found in sea plants, making avocados truly a unique vegetable, as it is one of the very few land plants to contain these fatty acids.

The high amounts of fatty acids in avocados, especially the oleic acids, can also help the body's digestive tracts transport molecules for fat to increase the body's absorption of nutrients that are fat soluble, like the carotenoids. These same fatty acids have also been shown to have benefits to the human heart, substantially decreasing the risk of heart disease as well.

All in all, people previously avoided avocados due to its reputation as a vegetable too high in fat, and that as a result it was an unhealthy vegetable to eat. But new studies within the last decade have proven that not only is that not the case, but that the reverse is actually true. Even though it is a true fact that an overwhelming majority of avocado calories come from fat, the fats in avocados are actually beneficial to human health.

Beets

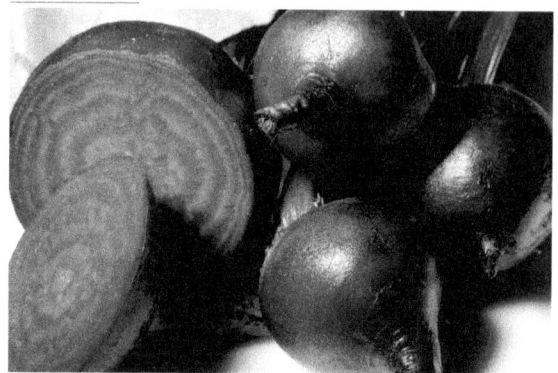

Beets contain large amounts of calcium, iron, magnesium and phosphorus. Beet roots posses many vitamins and minerals. Vitamins A, B and C are all present within the root.

Beets are colorful root vegetables that hold nutrient compounds that are extremely beneficial to defend against heart disease, colon cancer, and birth defects. First of all, the pigments that deliver beets their affluent colors are called betalains, of which there are two types: betacyanins and betaxanthins. Betacyanins are pigments that are red or violet in color. The most studied of the betacyanins are called betanin. Meanwhile, betaxanthins are colored yellow, but betacyanins are almost always the dominant color in red or purple colored beets. The reverse is true for yellow beats, where betaxanthins are by far the dominant pigment.

Many people rarely even thing about beets, with most people actually probably being turned away by them. If you are one of those people, its time to expand your horizons and become more open minded. Beets are incredibly healthy for your body, as well as among the best detoxifying foods. Beets have been scientifically proven to enhance a person's body physically, be a source of iron, and protect against cancer.

Even people who are aware of the health benefits of beets, however, often turn away from them because, well, they don't taste very well. However, people who do eat them gradually come to enjoy the taste of beets over time, much like cheeses or wines. In fact, many people who come to appreciate the numerous health benefits of beets end up eating it anyway and develop a love for them. Keep in mind as well, there are numerous ways you can cook beets. You can eat them chilled, slice them in a can (which involves absolutely no cooking by the way), or simply eat them naturally. But regardless of the way you choose to prepare your beets (just go online and you'll find hundreds of different ways you can prepare them), the nutritional health benefits of beets truly are spectacular; making them one of the more unexpected but also nutritious additions to the top ten super foods.

Ten Reasons to Eat Beets

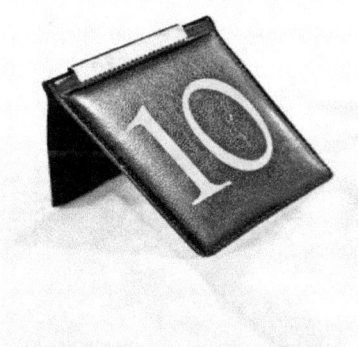

1. ZERO FAT

Beets do not have any Trans Fat or Saturated Fat. They are very low in calories and are very beneficial to those who have a sweet tooth, because beets have natural sugar.

2. Inexpensive to purchase

Being a root vegetable, beets do not cost much at your local grocer.

3. Energy

Beets are very high in healthful carbohydrates. They are considered a great source of energy. They body takes a while to digests the fibers and utilizes all the nutrients included.

4. Mineral Gold Mine

Beets posses many minerals and are high in sodium, magnesium, calcium, iron, and phosphorous. They promote healthy muscles and bone structure.

5. Prevents Cancer

Beets have been shown to reduce the risk of cancer, especially colon cancer. Beets posses Betacyanins, and that is the pigment that gives beets their red flavor. Betacyanins is the strongest known aid in preventing cancer.

6. Vitamins for Eye Sight

Beets come in many different colors. The colors that are orange, red, and purple are some of the flavonoids. The flavonoids are beneficial because they aid in the bodies regeneration. Vitamin A, C, and Niacin all reside in beets!

7. The Leaves are Edible!

Every part of the beet is edible. The leaves have been eaten since the Romans. Just drop your beets in the blender. They make ultimate smoothie addition.

8. Available Year Round

You can buy beets all year!

9. Heart Healthy

With beets being low in fat, very high in nutrients, very easy to digest, and full of beneficial compounds, it has also been shown that beets can help prevent heart disease.

10 Very Easy to Use!

Cook them, cut them, and eat them raw, you can use them in many ways.

A Beet Chips Recipe

With the use of a dehydrator or an oven, you can easily create crispy beet chips. This will allow you to absorb the many of the nutritional benefits…and enjoy the vegetable at the same time!

Beet tip: Salad Shreds

Use a grater and shred some beets into your salad! It will heighten the colors and increase your nutritional intake.

A Quick Juicing Recipe for Beets

For an easy and delicious juicing recipe add the following:

1. add   ½ Beet
2. add   2-3 Carrots
3. add   2 Apples
4. add   ½ Lime
5. Add   ¼ tbsp. knob of Ginger

A major benefit to beets is that they contain absolutely no saturated fats and absolutely no Trans fat. As a result, they are very low on calories. Beets are an excellent source of food for anybody who wants to fill their stomach to satisfy their hunger, without having to fill it with unhealthy foods (the very foods you're going to avoid, right?) Plain and simple, how could a person resist a food that doesn't do any harm to their body's health while also fulfilling their craving for sugar?

Beets are also high in carbohydrates, meaning that are an excellent source of instant energy. Of course, there are numerous other types of foods available on the market that are also high in carbohydrates (including some healthy foods), but unlike those foods, beets serve as fuel for your body and can provide instant energy.

Beets themselves hold high levels of phosphorous, calcium, iron, magnesium, and sodium, and Vitamin A and Vitamin C, thereby classifying them as a fiber food. They also contain folic acid that is a necessity for producing and maintaining new cells in the body. Most people are aware of this benefit of folic acid, but they instead take it as a herbal supplement, which not only is more expensive than beets but also don't have the additional nutritional values that beets have. After all, beets are food anyway. They're not a supplement. Why take a pill or a powder when you can eat real food?

The real benefits of beets, however, lie in the medical field. Scientific and medical studies have shown that beets serve as a protection against cancer, especially colon cancer, and helps protect the body against heart disease. So not only are you cleansing the inside of your body of unhealthy substances when you eat beets, you are also eating a safeguard against various threats to your body. Beets can also strengthen the gall bladder and the liver, and help to cleanse your bloodstreams. This is especially important, since blood travels throughout your entire body. Beets furthermore are useful in eliminating tumors, and reducing the chances of blood diseases and other forms of cancer such as leukemia.

As discussed before, there are literally hundreds of different ways you can prepare beets if you don't exactly fancy eating them plain or raw. They can be boiled, roasted, steamed, or sautéed, among other ways of preparation. However, one of the most popular ways to prepare beets is to make beet juice, which has a very powerful and strong taste. In order to make the taste of beet juice milder, you can blend it with other juices or beverages. You could potentially get the taste of apple or orange juice with the nutritional benefits of beets!

A slightly less relevant but nonetheless very interesting fact about beets is that they are naturally colorful (bright red, yellow, violet, etc.) and thus make for a superb decoration to adorn an already artistic looking meal. This can also be done with salads.

If price is an issue, it's good to know that beets or canned beats at least, are also very inexpensive. Most beets can be bought at your local grocery store for less than a dollar. All you have to do is put a few cans of beets in your refrigerator, and when you're hungry for something quick and cheap, you can eat them without having to cook.

Cranberries

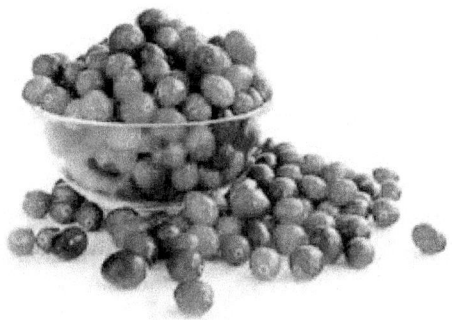

As you embark on your journey to detoxify your body, you will be
confronted with many different food options (a few of which we've
already gone over). However, hardly anyone knows that included in the
list of options for detoxifying foods are cranberries. That's right,
cranberries! The popular side dish on a traditional Thanksgiving dinner,
the cranberry juice stored on the shelves of grocery stores...it's a
detoxifying food source. If you thought that detoxifying your body
meant eliminating all forms of tasty (albeit unhealthy) foods, you're
wrong.

The fact that cranberries can prevent urinary tract infections (UTI's) isn't
exactly brand new news. It was already established far back in the 1900s
that cranberries can help prevent UTI's all the way back in the very early
1900s. However, these first reports were largely unreliable and sketchy.
Doctors at the time prescribed cranberries to patients on the rationale that
the acidic properties of them led to improving a person's urinary health.
New scientific research, however, has found that the real reason behind
cranberries aiding in enhancing urinary health is really the result of anti-
adhesive properties, not acidic properties. Phytochemicals in cranberries
avert bacteria from multiplying throughout the body. This alone
enhances urinary health. Certainly, multiple other types of fruits are
loaded with nutrients, anti-oxidants, and vitamins that improve bodily
health, but cranberries are unique as they are the only type of fruit that
contain these phytochemicals. Eat or drink as many of them as you will,

but grape juice, grapes, apple juice, apples, raisins or green tea will not prevent UTI's, as cranberries will. All you have to do is make a glass of cranberry juice a daily part of your diet (see, detox diets aren't that bad after all) and your urinary health is very likely to improve in a short period of time.

In addition, cranberries also contain calories are very nutritious and offer similar health benefits that can only be derived from cranberries. This is far different from the other juice or sweetened beverages you'll find at the grocery store.

Being UTI's, cranberries are also beneficial in that they can help to prevent cavities and substantially lower the risk of cancer. Cranberries slow down the production of harmful acids in your mouth, preventing bad bugs doing damage to your mouth and teeth (fewer trips to the dentist's office!)

Ten Reasons to eat Cranberries

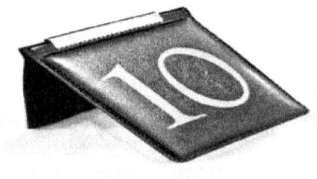

1. Cranberries has a high level of phytochemicals which is a substance found in plants that helps protect human cells. There have been over 150 phytochemicals identified in this berry so far.

2. Much research has been applied to learning the benefits that cranberries provide. One main attribute is that cranberries fight off bacteria and helps eliminate the bacteria found in urinary tract infections.

3. Cranberries also have antioxidant components, which help with the process of aging.

4. Even with the health of your heart, cranberries improve your artery walls helping fight off cardiovascular disease.

5. Current testing is being done because it is believed that since cranberries help protect human cells then they may be able to aid in the fight against cancer. The same is true for Alzheimer's disease.

6. It is proven that your body's defense mechanisms work better when cranberries are apart of your diet.

7. Cranberries contain a high amount of vitamin C and fiber.

8. Cranberries are a cholesterol free, fat free and low sodium food.

9. Because the antioxidant levels in cranberries, they support memory coordination and function.

10. Cranberries prevent plaque formation on the tooth enamel by interfering with the ability of another gram-negative bacterium, *Streptococcus mutans*, to stick to the surface. It thus helps prevent development of cavities.

Cranberries can also be a contributor to fighting cancer. While cranberries are definitely not a cure for cancer, they do lower the risk of it happening. Polyphenolics in cranberries inhibit the growth and abundant production of many different types of cancer, especially prostrate, lung, and colon cancer. This is because cranberries can restrain the growth of cancer cells by making harmful cells to die. This is a major impediment to cancer cells invading surrounding tissue anywhere in the body.

Whether you choose to drink a glass of cranberry juice every day, eat sweetened dried cranberries in the middle of a run, or add fresh cranberries to your next salad or meal, cranberries are without a doubt one of the more enjoyable detox foods. If you thought you would have to give up on all kinds of fruit juices entirely, you can make an exception for cranberry juice. And don't just follow the suggestions for preparing cranberries that are listed immediately above. Be creative and find some new ways to prepare them too. The possibilities are nearly endless.

Watercress

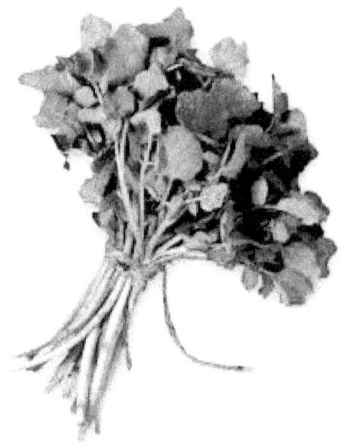

Believe it or not, but nearly one third of all cancers are either caused or partially caused because of poor diet choices or other related factors. As a result, there is no better time than now to make better choices in your daily diet to help combat the risk of cancer and other cancer related diseases in your body.

For many years, many people have held cruciferous vegetables in high regard for being 'anti-cancer.' Such vegetables include Brussels sprouts, cabbage, cauliflower and broccoli. No doubt, these vegetables when consumed do drastically help to reduce the risk of cancer as well as detoxify the body. But what many people don't know is that another cruciferous vegetable, watercress, has displayed even greater potential in helping to prevent and/or reduce the risk of cancer. At the same time, watercress's offers the same healthy green vegetable substance that it is necessary for a healthy daily diet.

How does watercress manage to lead to an even greater reduction in the risk of cancer than other green vegetable plants? It's because watercress has the ability to increase the level of antioxidants in the bloodstream of the human body. This protects DNA molecules against damage, while also lowering the risk of breast, prostrate, or colon cancer from infecting the human body. Watercress is a first rate source of Vitamin A, Vitamin C, and Vitamin K. These antioxidant vitamins are also a crucial micronutrient for bone health, as well as a rich source of carotenoids nutrients that help protect cardiovascular health and vision.

Most cruciferous green vegetables are renowned for holding phytochemicals that hydrolyze to produce isothiocyanates, which has been studied some time for its anti-cancer effects. Daily intake of these compounds in a person's diet reveals to be one of the principle reasons that Watercress is so effective at reducing the risk of cancer: head, colorectal, head, neck, breast, lung and prostrate, primarily. These compounds have also been shown be a rich dietary source of nasturtium, a compound that provokes the emission of carcinogens in the body.

Ten Reason to eat more Watercress

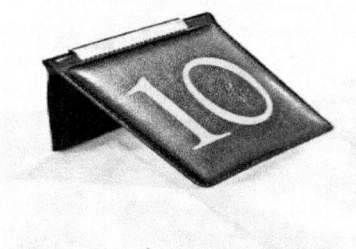

1. Full of ANTIOXIDANTS

The Lutein and Zeaxanthin in watercress are reasons to eat watercress because they help maintain clear skin. Lutein plays a part in eye health also. Make watercress a part of your salad!

2. Aphrodisiac

One of the best reasons to eat watercress is for its aphrodisiac properties. In GREECE for generations it has been passed down to conceive children.

3. It can be a hangover cure

Blend watercress with your favorite fruit juice to help alleviate the symptoms.

4. BRAIN FOOD

In Greece, watercress was not just used to help with children to aid in the intellectual growth.

5. Very Low Calories

Only 18 calories per serving!

6. Fight Cancer

Watercress, along with broccoli, cauliflower, rocket, cabbage, sprouts and radishes are believed to contain properties that can fight against cancer.

7. Breast Cancer Prevention

British scientists are conducting research into watercress and the prevention of Breast cancer. So far watercress has reduced the cancer in the test subjects by 35%!

8. Provide a great source of Beta-Carotene

Watercress is packed with beta-carotene. Beta-Carotene is a substance, which helps to keep your eyes and skin healthy and fresh.

9. VITAMINS

Of course, watercress is a great source of many key vitamins, which are crucial to children's development. Watercress can provide iron, manganese, zinc and calcium, as well as vitamins E, C, B1, B6 and K.

10. PREGNANCY HELP

Another of the reasons why watercress is good for you is because of the vital vitamins – such as folic acid – This is very helpful with the fetus.

Watercress

Even crude watercress has found to provide a significant defense against colon cancer cells and the three steps of the carcinogenic process. These three steps, in respective order, are initiation, proliferation, and metastasis. Compounds from watercress inhibit the activity of enzymes that progress cancers by breaking apart barriers in body that were in turn supposed to inhibit the expanding bad tumors. These same watercress compounds can also repress enveloping breast cancer cell lines, as well as restrain inflammatory compounds that cause chronic inflammation and cancer during cellular activity.

We've all grown up knowing that eating your green vegetables was healthy, but did you grow up know they were actually this beneficial and nutritious for your body? Watercress is a natural source of lutein and zeaxanthin, two carotenoids that have been found to be beneficial for the heart and eyes. Daily intake of these carotenoids in your daily diet will also lead to a much lower risk of macular eye degeneration, the most abundant source of blindness in adults. Just one cup of raw watercress a day will get you nineteen hundred mcg of lutein and zeaxanthin, meaning that eating raw watercress alone will reduce your chances of becoming blind or gradually losing vision later in life.

These same carotenoids have also found to offer protective defenses for the body's cardiovascular system. People who have high levels of lutein and zeaxanthin in their body's blood stream are likely to have a lesser chance of hardening your arteries in the neck, at last a substantially lesser chance than people with lower levels of these two carotenoids in their blood levels. Because of this protection of the cardiovascular system, people with high levels of carotenoids in their blood levels are also less likely to undergo a heart attack later in their life. See how healthy eating your green vegetables really is?

Well now that you do know all of the benefits that your green vegetables and watercress in particular, have for your body, the next question is how you would prepare watercress to be a tasty part of your daily diet as well. This question mainly comes up because, granted, no one's going to want to suffice on raw watercress for the rest of his or her lives.

All you have to really do to prepare watercress is to trim the stems, and then rinse it in cold water and set out to dry or use a paper towel. Then, you can either use it immediately or store in a packed container in the cooler or the refrigerator. You can use watercress in sandwiches, salads, soup, as a garnish, or pretty much any other recipe where you would have used lettuce. This means you can prepare watercress to be fried, steamed, etc. But whether you choose to prepare your watercress raw or cook, it will still have the same anti-cancer effects no matter what.

Overall, we've always known that eating our green vegetables was always the most healthy part of our diet, but more recent scientific and medical studies conducted have shown that no leafy, green vegetable has as much nutritional or health related value as much as watercress. Watercress is an abundant natural source for Vitamins A, C and K, as well as containing compounds that can fight the risk of cancer, as well as other health related topics. Plus, the two carotenoids found in watercress, lutein and zeaxanthin, has also been found to have enormous benefits on eye and cardiovascular health.

Cilantro

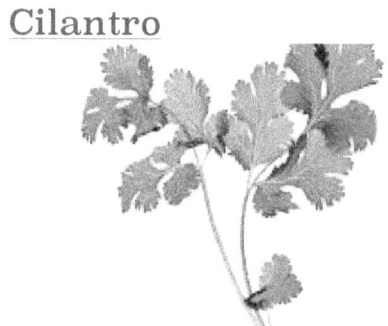

Cilantro is a Mediterranean herb that is popular as a component of savory dishes for traditional as well as more modern meals. In use since the times of the Ancient Greeks and Romans, Cilantro has also been found to carry notable chemical compounds that can prevent or inhibit diseases and promote health. The clean and anti-septic properties of cilantro can be found in the leaves, roots and stems of the plant. Cilantro is a rich, natural source for vitamins and anti-oxidants, including Vitamin C, that offer a wide variety of health benefits, as we shall very soon see.

Fact: Cilantro may be used to treat urinary tract infection.

Cilantro has been found to have benefits for cardiovascular health. On basic terms, there are two types of cholesterol: bad cholesterol and good cholesterol. Bad cholesterol is widely regarded to be the LDL cholesterol, while good cholesterol is regarded to be HDL cholesterol. Cilantro is free of cholesterol, but it is also a rich natural source for anti-oxidants, Vitamin C, dietary fibers and oils, which help lower LDL cholesterol levels and increase HDL cholesterol levels. This helps to dissolve cholesterol built up in and disrupting the arteries, greatly minimalizing the risk of heart disease.

Fact: Cilantro is considered a member of the carrot family.

Cilantro has also been found to lower blood sugar. This may at first seem obvious since cilantro can lower LDL cholesterol, however it can also work to decrease hypertension by lowering blood pressure. Cilantro is a natural source of magnesium, calcium, manganese, potassium, iron, and low levels of sodium. This make up of cilantro is what allows it to help your body control your heart rate and lower your blood pressure. Iron is also especially critical for the production of red blood cells, and manganese is also important as a co-factor for enzymes that are anti-oxidant. Because cilantro can lower blood sugar and blood pressure, it also greatly reduces the risk of acquiring diabetes. If you already have diabetes however, cilantro herbs can still regulate it and keep your blood sugar levels stable.

10 Healthy Cilantro Benefits

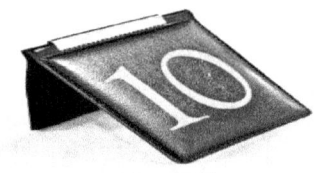

1. Nutritive

Cilantro is a good source of dietary fiber, magnesium, and iron. It is rich in Flavonoids and phytonutrients. It is also an excellent source of antioxidants.

2. Digestive Aide

Prevents flatulence and can help settle a stomach. Cilantros will also sooth nausea in the body. Cilantro aids the digestive system produce digestive enzymes, and also produces more digestive juices.

3. An Anti-inflammatory

Can alleviate inflammatory conditions in the body. Minor swelling and arthritis are some examples.

4. Chelation aide

Aides in the removal of heavy metals from the body and help remove toxicity.

5. Helps the Liver Functions

Will lower the bad cholesterol and supports the good cholesterol.

6. Posses anti-bacterial Properties

Studies have shown it to be very effective against Salmonella bacteria. Can also help to relieve diarrhea.

7. Aides with insulin Secretion

Can be an affective aide in fight and preventing diabetes.

8. Immune boosting properties

With all the vitamins and minerals within, it is great at boosting ones immunity.

9. Can acts as an expectorant

10. Will stimulate the endocrine glands

Cilantro can also help to relax your anxiety, largely due to the fact that cilantro can help to loosen up your muscles and calming the nerves. This helps relieve the stress in your body, and along with that all of the harmful effects that stress has. Not only does stress weaken you physically, it also weakens you mentally and disrupts your ability to think clearly and comprehensively. Sometimes all it takes to get back on track in our lives is to relieve all the stress, and cilantro is an excellent way to do that. All you need to do is drink some cilantro juice; it's filled with Vitamin B allowing you to clear your mind and calm down. In addition, since cilantro can help you to reduce stress by relaxing your muscles and nerves, it can also help you sleep longer and better.

Cilantro has also been found to help relieve digestion and nausea problems to aid in preventing diarrhea and vomiting. Producing digestive enzymes in your digestive system does this. The digestive system, as a result impeded flatulence and related substances that can result from an uneasy stomach. The herbs in cilantro can as a result not only stimulate digestion, but also lead to making your liver healthier via anti-oxidant properties and using fiber to help relieve gastrointestinal problems.

However, one of the real gems of cilantro herbs as a detox food source is that it can remove heavy metal substances from within your body. Wait a second, how did heavy metals enter your body in the first place? Usually heavy metal substances enter the body via eating non-organic food, like fish in aluminum foil, or using deodorant, smoking cigarettes, or having metal fillings your teeth. These heavy metals can cause serious health issues like cancer, brain impediment, and diseases relating to the lung, heart, and kidneys, or weakening the bone structure. Cilantro can assemble mercury from the brain and nervous system by extracting it from fat tissues and sending it into the blood stream. This greatly aids in reducing the risk of mercury poisoning, which is toxic to the body and especially to the blood stream. Cilantro is able to accomplish this via chemical compounds within the herb.

Yes, deodorant can be a source of getting these deadly heavy metal substances in your body. Does that mean that you can no longer use deodorant? Of course not! If you want to avoid deodorant entirely though, you can turn to natural sources of it. Yes, cilantro herbs are considered to be a natural deodorant, only it's an internal deodorant in that it detoxifies your body from the inside out. It removes toxins and bacteria from your body that would band together in your armpits and feet. This is because of chlorophyll contained in the cilantro herbs that impede bacteria due to high oxygen levels. This essentially means that you can deodorize your body from the inside out...and smell great at the same time.

Cilantro also contains anti-oxidant properties that protect the body's cells against oxidation. This delays the ageing process of the body and prevents diseases that typically come with age, such as cancer, diabetes, Alzheimer's, heart issues, and degeneration of the bone structure. Think about it. Cilantro cannot only make you look younger; it can make you feel younger too!

Cilantro holds a compound called dodecenal, which is an anti bacteria compound that can kill bacteria and prevent bacteria poisoning. This can enhance oral health and help prevent and treat small pox, in addition to relieving diarrhea or vomiting, among other infections caused by bacteria invasions.

Cilantro can also help with a wide variety of other health treatments. It can aid in weight loss by reducing fats in the body, especially for obese people. Since cilantro is a rich natural source of vitamins and minerals such as iron and magnesium, it can also function the nervous system properly and strengthen your bones. Just chewing a few cilantro leaves would be extremely helpful for you if you suffer from asthma or bronchitis, and the oil from cilantro herbs can help in curing any mouth ulcers you may or may not have.

Last but certainly not least, cilantro also has many benefits for the skin and hair. We all long for attractive looking skin, but it takes more than just outside oils and substances to make our skin look good. Believe it or not, but the biggest reason that can lead to your skin looking good comes from the inside of our body. Your body requires nutrition to maintain good health, and that includes your skin as well. So before we get into the details of how cilantro can aid your skin, it is important you know that how crucial it is to maintain a proper diet, and limit exposure to UV rays or difficult chemical treatments.

That said, cilantro juice is an effective treatment for blackheads and/or acne on your face. If you blend approximately one teaspoon of cilantro juice with approximately one teaspoon of lime juice and apply it to blackheads and acne on your face, and then leave it undisturbed for about an hour, you should start to see some results. Largely for the same reasons, cilantro can also act as a treatment for more serious skin disorders by serving as an anti septic and anti fungal treatment for skin disorders such as eczema, dermatitis, and small pox. Cilantro can also absorb extra oil from your face, so if you have oily skin all you need to do is apply some cilantro juice and hot water to your face and you should look better in no time! You can do this same thing if you have dark lips; simply applying warm water with cilantro to your lips can make them lighten up in color quickly too.

As discussed above, cilantro can cause anti ageing due to several anti-oxidants that prevent the skin cells from being damaged, and that not only can you look younger as you age, but you can even feel younger as well. Vitamin A, a fat-soluble vitamin and anti-oxidant, can be used for upholding healthy mucus membranes and skin. Meanwhile, Vitamin C can prevent any signs of ageing like sagging skin, pigmentation, and even wrinkles.

Cilantro also fights hair loss. After all, all you really need to do to maintain a good amount of hair on your head is make sure you get a good supply of nutrients from your daily diet into your system (for most people, at least...). Cilantro can help you keep hair on your head as well. This is because that cilantro contains vitamins and proteins that help in growing you hair, fighting existing hair loss, and encouraging new hair growth if you're already balding. All you need to do is make a paste from cilantro leaves by mixing its juice with warm water. If you apply this to your head before shampooing your head in the shower for about two to three weeks, you should witness fast and effective results. You can find the same results by permeating your hair with a powder from cilantro seeds or rinsing your hair by boiling cilantro leaves in water (though you may want to cool down the now boiled water before applying it to your head).

Citrus Fruit

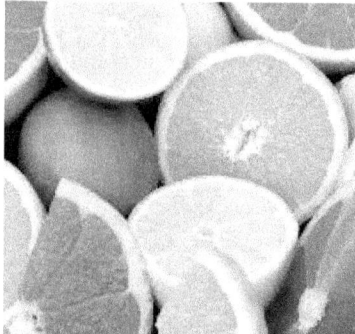

Citrus fruits have always been appreciated as being part of a nutritious and healthy. But only do most citrus fruits taste extremely good, they are very good for the body as well. They are a rich, natural source of minerals, vitamins, and dietary fibers. These are critical not only for growth and development of the body, but for the nutritional maintenance of it as well. But not only are citrus fruits rich sources of minerals and vitamins, they can also help to prevent many different types of diseases.

The main nutrient contained in citrus fruits is carbohydrate (carbs). Citrus holds carbs such as glucose, sugars, fructose and sucrose, in addition to citric acid (hence the name 'citrus fruit'). Citrus fruits also hold non-starch polysaccharides (NSP), such as dietary fibers, which is important to enhancing health. The most common type of dietary fibers found in citrus fruits are pectin and cellulose. These fibers hold nutrients that are water soluble and slow down absorption and digestion, which in turn reduces the rate of glucose intake following bodily consumption of carbs and stopping a surge of glucose levels in the blood stream.

Citrus fruit can also strengthen ligaments, tendons, skin, bones, and blood vessels, as well as heal wounds and repair tissues. This is because of the high levels of Vitamin C found in citrus fruits that are also soluble in water and form collagen, a large component of connective tissues throughout the body. Without the strengthening of these tissues, Vitamin C essentially decreases resulting in Vitamin C deficiency. Plain and simple, Vitamin C is extremely important to the body and by aiding in the treatment of stress levels, as well as reduce symptoms of the common cold.

One of the main reasons however, of why Vitamin C is such an important detox food is because of its anti-oxidant properties. Anti-oxidants basically can prevent cell damage done by 'radical' molecules that oxidize protein, DNA and fatty acids. Radical molecule damage also goes beyond just oxidization by leading to some more advanced diseases throughout the body, including heart and lung disease, decrease in vision, and a higher risk of cancer. That's why that including citric fruits, such as lemons and oranges, into your daily diet will already be a huge help to reduce the risks of these diseases from ever happening in your lifetime.

Another important vitamin found in citrus fruits is folate, which is also soluble in water. Folate is critical for producing new cells and growing them, aiding in DNA and RNA production and growing red blood cells, preventing a deficiency of red blood cells that can unleash a whole new array of potential health diseases. Generally speaking, a daily intake of anywhere from two hundred to four hundred mcg of folate is what it is needed for seeing any real progress and preventing future diseases.

Ten Reasons to eat Citrus Fruits Everyday

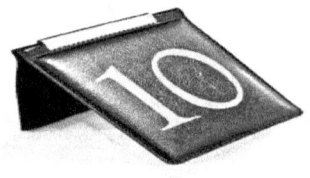

1. They will Boosts your immunity

A single citrus fruit can meet more than 100% of your daily requirement of Vitamin C. This vital nutrient helps improve your immunity and fighting off diseases.

2. Very Good for your skin

Aging of your skin is inevitable, but citrus fruits are packed with antioxidants and Vitamin C, which slows down the process and makes you look younger than you really are.

3. Great for your eye health

Our eyes suffer from damage, as we grow older. Citrus fruits are rich in nutrients like Vitamin A, Vitamin C and potassium, which are great for your eye health.

4. Will help Prevent heart disease

Citrus fruits have flavonoids like hesperidin, which reduces cholesterol and prevents your arteries from getting blockage. This can help prevent heart disease.

5. Helps with brain development

Folate and folic acid present in citrus fruit promote brain development. These nutrients also make citrus fruit a healthy for pregnant woman.

6. Helps Prevent cancer

Research has shown that a compound called D – limonene present in citrus fruit can prevent various types of cancer like lung cancer, breast cancer, skin cancer, etc. Citrus fruit's antioxidants and Vitamin C help promote your body's immunity, which helps in fighting cancer cells and other various diseases.

7. Prevents stomach ulcers

Citrus Fruits are a very good source of fiber. Fiber keeps your stomach and intestines healthy. A diet rich in fiber provides the best intestinal and stomach care available.

8. Improves your sperm quality

Citrus Fruit's antioxidants and Vitamin C improves the quality and motility of your sperm. This keeps you fertile.

9. Great for someone who is diabetic

Diabetes prevents the body from absorbing glucose. The beta cells present in the pancreas either fail to produce insulin or the body's cells are unable to respond to the insulin produced. Citrus fruits are high in fiber and have a high glycemic index that makes it a good food option for diabetics.

10. Help Prevent hair loss

Citrus Fruit's are high Vitamin C content which is required for producing collagen. The collagen is responsible for keeping your hair together.

Citrus fruits also contain high levels of potassium, a critical mineral for maintaining the water and acid balance of the body. Potassium is also an electrolyte that transmits nerve impulses to the muscles, aids in muscle contraction, and maintains normal levels of blood pressure. A good rule of thumb is to include approximately two thousand mg's of potassium in your daily diet. While this may seem a lot, and while eating less than this amount will in no way lead to potassium deficiencies (which are already rare), it is generally recommended that you try to eat as much potassium as you can daily, especially in ratio to high levels of sodium intake, in order to prevent diseases. Approximately one orange alone with provide you with two hundred and thirty five mg of potassium. There are other sources of potassium as well, however, so you don't simply have to continuously eat eight or nine oranges every day.

A naturally occurring compound found in citrus fruit is phytochemicals, which have a very important effect on the body. They can defend against numerous types of chronic diseases, the most deadly being heart related diseases and cancer. As we continue to expand our knowledge of phytochemicals, we will continue to learn and understand the role they play in benefiting the human body. What we know so far, however, is that phytochemicals do have anti-oxidation properties, differentiate cells, lead to increased activity of enzymes that detoxify carcinogens, and that the only way we can truly intake a regular, varied mix of phytochemicals is through the consumption of citrus fruits, among other plant based foods.

Blueberries

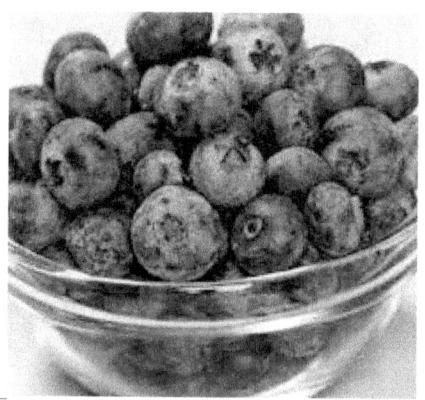

Believe it or not, but blueberries are indeed a detoxification food. They hold anti-oxidants that neutralize 'radical' molecules found in the body that can lead to cancer, heart and/or lung disease, or ageing conditions. Blueberries may be small, little tasty fruits, but they are also small but mighty health enhancers. Blueberries are also very low in fat, clocking it at only about eighty calories per cup, and are packed with dietary fiber.

They are a rich, natural source of manganese, can strengthen bone structure, and convert carbohydrates (carbs) and fats into sources of energy. They have also been found to improve brain healthy and combat infections in the urinary tract, making them a possible cancer fighter.

Ten Reasons to eat Blueberries everyday

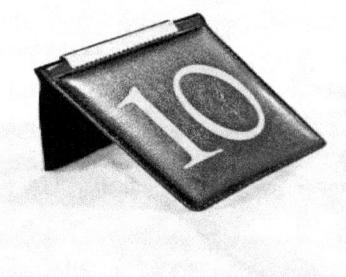

1) To help Fatten your stomach

Blueberries have catechins, which are natural antioxidants. Catechins are plentiful in blueberries; activate your fat-burning genes in the stomach area. That's right, eating blueberries can help you get that 6-pack!

2) Your brain health

Blueberries contain phytonutrients called proanthocyanidins, which help protect your brains watery and fatty tissues against damage.

3) Help keep your youthful appearance.

The same proanthocyanidins that help protect your brain can help keep your skin looking young. If you want to eliminate those wrinkles, eat blueberries.

4) Helps your memory and motor skills.

Studies have shown that when blueberry extract people have better memories versus the test subjects not given the extract.

5) Fights against cancer.

Blueberries are full of ellagic acid. Ellagic acid has been proven to be a cancer fighter.

6) Helps with allergies.

Blueberries include a lot of quercetin. Quercetin is a powerful phytonutrient. It will reduce the severity of your allergies.

7) Natural Aspirin

Blueberries put salicylic acid into your system. Salicylic acid is the natural form of aspirin.

8) Helps with your mood.

Eating blueberries contain dopamine. Dopamine is a natural neurotransmitter that tells your mind it feels good.

9) Great for your diet.

Blueberries are full of a lot of the things your body (and brain) need to function properly: iron, magnesium, potassium, riboflavin, niacin, folate and vitamins C and E. Full plate of all the goodies.

10) Taste great with natural sugar

Blueberries taste great and are great for you.

One thing to know about blueberries is that they contain tons of Vitamin C. Literally tons. Okay, not 'literally tons' but you get the point; they carry a lot of Vitamin C, especially for such a little fruit. Approximately one serving of blueberries alone will get you twenty five percent of the average human body's daily needs of Vitamin C. Vitamin C in this case is important because it leads to healthier gums in the mouth, a healthier immune system, and decreasing the risk of eye conditions.

Blueberries can also improve health of the heart. Currently, cardiovascular disease is the number one cause of death in the United States and a huge public health concern. Heart disease in the first place can be caused by a number of different factors, including but certainly not limited to high levels of blood pressure, blood sugar and obesity. New scientific studies though have revealed that blueberries may actually reduce the risk of heart diseases, and furthermore can actually build up cardiovascular health. People who eat more blueberries as part of their daily diet than other people are far less likely to develop a lung or heart disease at some later point in their life.

Blueberries can also help to reduce the risk of developing cancer, and in this case it's all in the color of the blueberries, only literally this time. Anthocyanins are what give blueberries their blue color, but they also help to improve cardiovascular health and defend the body against radical molecules that can be a major cause of developing cancer in the body, especially prostate cancer. Plain and simple, blueberries have been found to be a means of preventing, or at least of substantially lowering the risk of, cancer. It's funny to think that it's the literal blue color of blueberries that leads to this, but hey, facts are facts.

Blueberries have also been found to fight urinary tract infections (UTI's). UTI's form and grow inside the urinary tract. They are caused by bacteria and can cause a wide range of potential infections. Symptoms include a strong, unrelenting urge to urinate often, as well as urine that smells poorly (not that urine doesn't already smell poorly, just it would smell even more so). Overall, UTI's are far more common in women than in men, with one in every two or one half, of woman having at least one UTI in their lifetime. Blueberries can fight UTI's in largely the same way that cranberries do. Both blueberries and cranberries fight UTI's with compounds that stop bacteria from sticking to bladder walls. This is done because they hold substances that impede bacteria from binding to the bladder tissue on the walls. Eating blueberries as a part of your daily diet will greatly aid in reducing symptoms and fighting UTI's.

Last but not least, blueberries have been found to boost brain health, by reducing the risk of memory loss. It may be hard to believe that you can protect your mental comprehension and ability later on in life just by eating a handful of blueberries every day, but you can.

Overall, blueberries are an excellent detox food. These small but mighty fruits fight urinary tract infections, the risk of developing prostrate cancer, and improving the health of the heart.

Cabbage

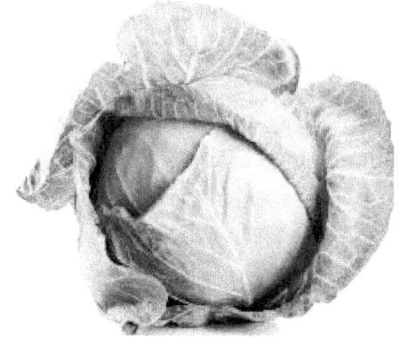

What turns many people away from cabbage isn't because it's tasty or because people don't know it's nutritious. It's because cabbage isn't exactly the most thrilling or attractive food on the aisle at the grocery store. While it's true that cabbage isn't the most appealing food to most people, it still hides a load of important minerals, vitamins and nutrients that help to fight diseases and help to prevent cancer, decrease cholesterol, and mend ulcers.

Ten Reason to eat cabbage everyday

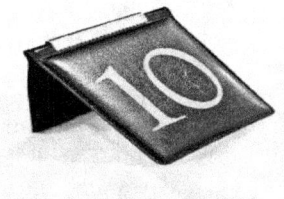

1. Cabbage is low in calorie, high in fiber and has zero fat.

2. Cabbage is very high in iron content.

3. Cabbage has a tremendous amount of Vitamin K.

4. Cabbage is filled with powerful antioxidants.

5. Cabbage is one of the best anti-inflammatory foods.

6. Cabbage is wonderful for cardiovascular support.

7. Cabbage is very high in Vitamin A.

8. Cabbage is a great source for Vitamin C.

9. Cabbage is very high in calcium.

10. Cabbage is one of the best detox super foods.

Cabbage comes from a family of vegetables called Brassica vegetables. This family of vegetables includes cauliflower, kale, broccoli, and Brussels sprouts...and yes, cabbage too. While there are nutritional heath benefits to each of these mentioned vegetables in the Brassica family (among others), none are as nutritious as cabbage. Cabbage provides number of health benefits and from all forms of cabbage as well. Green, red, white, and savoy cabbages that are all offered at your local grocery store (or should be offered, at least) contain the same nutritional values. After all, cabbage is sometimes considered to be the number one 'health food' due to the cabbage soup diet, a stern (and poor tasting) plan where you have to eat up to fifteen pounds worth of cabbage in a soup per week. While this is certainly one way to lose weight, among other health advantages, there are other, better ways to prepare and eat cabbage too.

Facts: cabbage has anti-inflammatory properties that can help with arthritis.

Cabbage is an incredible source of fiber, with raw cabbage alone being proven to be a cure to stomach ulcers. However, this alone does not discredit other vegetable members of the Brassica family, such as broccoli or Brussels sprouts, both of which contain high levels of fiber as well.

Cabbage, especially red cabbage, is also full of anti-oxidants. These anti-oxidants can help to reduce inflammation, defend against cancer and some of the causes of it in the body, and enhance cognition function.

When you eat cabbage, you also eat lower amounts of cholesterol. Cabbage is a natural reducer of cholesterol, which prevents bile-absorbing fat from a meal.

Cabbage also holds compounds known as glucosinolates that are sulfur based and have anti carcinogenic properties. These glucosinolates turn into compounds known as isothiocynates that have been shown to impede the growth of cancer cells, and reduce the risk of cancer as a whole.

So while cabbage can provide just as, if not more, impressive nutritional qualities and benefits as other green vegetables, you may want to consider using cabbage as an alternate green vegetables in recipes and meals, instead of other green vegetables such as lettuce. A good rule of thumb to remember is that deeply colored vegetables, such as dark green, red, purple, etc. contain more anti oxidants. This would include cabbage, since they come in a wider variety of deep colors. You basically get to take you pick based on your favored color!

Unfortunately, a major downside to cabbage is that the chemical compounds within it that hold such impressive nutritional qualities and benefits get broken down when affected by heat, or when it is cooked. This can be remedied however, by either eating cabbage completely or mostly raw, or cooking it lightly by either steaming or sautéing it to avoid as much heat on it as possible and to capitalize on the health benefits of it.

However you may not want to include purely raw cabbage with every meal, as despite the immense nutritional values and benefits of cabbage that we've discussed too much cabbage can actually be a bad thing for your body. This is another downside to cabbage, as an excess of it raw can lead to hormonal imbalance or deficiency of iodine levels in your body, by impeding your body's capability to absorb the iodine in the first place. Fortunately, this drawback is largely remedied purely by cooking cabbage, and should not discourage you from trying it as part of your daily meal.

Fortunately, a major pro to cabbage is price. If you are on a budget, you should know first that cabbage is rather cheap; stores well in that it can be kept in the refrigerator or cooler for up to two weeks, and are generally available throughout most of the year in grocery and market stores. This makes it an all round nutritious and economical detox food to turn to

Tahini

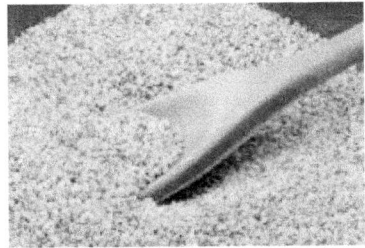

Also known as sesame butter, and long a popular food as a part of Asian cooking, Tahini has long had a reputation as a nutritious food only available in health stores. That's not entirely true; sure, Tahini is found in health stores, but it's also very much ground in your average grocery

or market store as well. Tahini is a light pasted produced from the kernel of sesame seeds that have been compressed and compacted, hence the term 'sesame butter.' The outside cases of the sesame seeds are detached as the crushed seeds are grounded into a chunky paste.

Facts: Tahini is a major component of hummus

Tahini is indeed a very nutritious and detoxifying food. While Tahini is very rich in fat, only roughly ten percent of this fat is saturated fat; the rest are fatty acids, or 'good' fats, that are critical for good health. Tahini holds high quality amounts of Omega 3 and 6 fatty acids, so only one table spoon of Tahini holds roughly eight five calories. Of those eighty five calories, about sixty five of them come from the 'good' fat, containing a few grams of protein and dietary fiber each. As a result, Tahini is an excellent, natural source of a wide variety of healthy vitamins and minerals including, but not limited to, Vitamin B, magnesium, phosphorous, copper, manganese and iron.

10 health benefits of tahini:

1. **Tahini is very rich in phosphorus, lecithin, potassium and iron**

2. **It is one of the best sources of Methionine. Methionine helps the Liver with detoxifying the body.**

3. **It provides as one of the best sources of calcium available.**

4. Loaded with Vitamins: E, B1, B2, B3, B5, and B15

5. Promotes Cell Growth

6. Helps with Prevention of Anemia

7. Very beneficial for Healthy Skin and enhancing muscle tone.

8. Very high source of protein. Made of 20% complete protein.

9. Very easy to digest due to a high alkaline content.

10. Very high in the good fat (unsaturated fat)

Tahini has been found to be beneficial towards cardiovascular health. It has been shown through scientific research that Tahini is an excellent source of phytosterols, compounds that reduce LDL, otherwise known as 'bad' cholesterol, in the body's blood stream. Tahini also holds dietary fibers called sesamin and sasamolin, which also can inhibit LDL cholesterol as well as high levels of blood pressure. The seeds in Tahini themselves are an excellent natural source of magnesium that loosens up blood vessels and in turn lowers the blood pressure. This allows blood circulation to flow easier and thus supports healthy cardiovascular health. Fatty acids in Tahini can also help to reduce hypertension and improve health of the heart and lungs do to a special hormone called prostaglandins.

Tahini can also help to improve the brain. Tahini contains high levels of Omega 3 and 6 acids that support healthy nervous tissues and enhance the cognitive and emotional health functions of the brain. These same fatty acids, in addition to the manganese contained in the sesame paste, can also inhibit the potential progression of Alzheimer's disease and harsh memory loss.

Tahini also holds a lot of anti-oxidant properties. This is because Tahini is an excellent natural source for copper, a mineral that contains properties that are anti inflammatory in composition. This, in addition to the high levels of Omega 3 and 6 fatty acids, helps to relieve pain and swelling in the event of arthritis. Copper can also help make easy the anti oxidant properties of enzymes within the immune system. The phytonutrients contained within Tahini defends the liver from any form of oxidative damage. Tahini also holds high levels of magnesium that relieves asthma as well.

Last but not least, Tahini has been shown to have benefits for vascular and respiratory health. This is because the sesame seeds contained in Tahini hold an impressive portion of the human body's daily necessity for the mineral magnesium. Magnesium inhibits constriction of the air ways to help prevent the potential onset of asthma, enhances blood vessels and blood circulation, and also helps to lower blood pressure, improving health of the heart and of the circulatory system.

PART 2

What Happened? Weight Loss Stops

You seem to have a clear vision. You want to lose weight as quickly as you can. Perhaps there is an upcoming event that has given you the urge to shed the pounds. It all starts off well. You put your plan into place, figure out how you will lose the weight and are so eager to get started. You're inspired and feel confident in your abilities to quickly get the weight off. Most people who want to lose weight start off with a positive attitude and a plan that is all lay on the line. The plan is fixed to a "T" and all seems so clear in your visions.

So, with all of the eagerness of a lion you start your diet, begin exercising more often and are making progress. You are on track and all seems well. You are losing weight, you feel great. People are complimenting you and telling you how great you look. You're happy and feel so much better inside. Nothing in this world could be better!

And then it happens... you hit the plateau. It seems that no matter what you do or how hard you try, no more weight will come off. You're stuck at the same weight and nothing is happening. You're doing all of the same things that you've been doing, but nothing comes about from it. What could be going wrong? Why this sudden stop when all was going so well?

This is very frustrating. You have come so very far in your weight loss efforts and now nothing is happening. It isn't just a few days; this can go on for weeks on end. All of the positive energy that you had flowing through you is now gone, and you do not feel like you'll ever again meet one of your weight loss goals. You are ready to throw in the towel; ready to give up and call it quits. It is apparent that you're doomed to be bigger than the average person and always keep those extra pounds on you.

Why does this happen? When everything is going so well, all of a sudden this plateau sneaks out of nowhere and throws you for a loop, as well as all of the great hinges that you were trying to do. You are confused worried and wondering what to do next when this happens to you, and with good reason, of course.

Relax. Take a deep breath and understand that you're not doing anything wrong. These plateaus are normal, and almost everyone who is trying to lose weight will experience them. It is difficult to deal with such events, but knowing it is not caused by something that you are doing wrong (obviously you're doing things right since you have accomplished so much thus far) and, this too shall pass. As hard as it might seem right now, you can overcome the hurdle and continue to shed the pounds, if you can remain positive and continue to do what you have been doing. What is important at this point is to understand that they happen and are very normal, and that you can overcome them with just a bit of desire and effort to do so.

Understanding the Plateau

A weight loss plateau is a time frame that your body stays the same weight even though you are still following your diet to specifications and participating in exercise on a regular basis. The length of time varies from person to person, but despite the fallback it doesn't mean that your efforts have gone to waste. For most people it is considered a plateau when there has been no change in the weight for a period of 3 weeks or more. It is common to see some weight steadiness as your attempt to lose those pounds.

Now, it is perfectly common to see fluctuations in your weight, especially if you are an individual who finds themself weighing on the scales on a frequent basis. If you do it several times per day, you may even notice that each time you step on the scale there is a 2 to 5 pound difference in the previous amount that you weighed. This is normal, and oftentimes associated with water retention. But, when the waft remains within this consistency for several weeks, it is considered the plateau.

A few things to keep in mind about the weight-loss plateau:

Weight Loss, Weight Slow-Downs

This is a fact of life: the more weight you lose; the more weight loss will slow down. If you lose 1% of your body fat each week, you're losing about 2 pounds of fat each week, too. Once you start to lose weight the amount of body fat that is coming off of the body is less, so you cannot lose as much. The more weight, the less that is coming off since you are now much leaner than before. It is simple mathematics.

Plateaus are Common

You should make plans to deal with the plateau at the same time as you are making plans to lose weight and your approach to doing them. While it may seem as if the plateau is a hurdle or an obstacle in your weight loss endeavors, it is actually a sign that you are doing something right and if you are able to make just a few changes you will be able to continue to make those great accomplishments. You should plan for them to happen as you begin to lose weight, and it might even be more than one of them that you will experience. If it were that easy to lose weight there would be no one with weight problems!

Use Your Time Wisely

The weight loss plateau may be difficult to deal with, but it is also a great time to think things through and take a clear look at your approach to losing weight. Should you change the way that you are doing things, considering the fact you're not smaller than before and have already made great accomplishments? These are just some of the things to consider as you face the challenges of the plateau.

Some people will also face those great hurdles in their weight loss efforts because they are not going about things in a healthy way. You cannot start to see the results and then start on your whirlwind lifestyle all over again. You must be ready to commit to the new and improved lifestyle. There are a number of consequences that come with unhealthy dieting practicing's. Let's take a look at some of those.

1. Binge Eating

Unhealthy dieting can result in feelings of food deprivation. If you cut your calories excessively, eliminate all of the foods you call your favorites and eat very little food that delivers much needed nutrition, the consequences are often the need to make up for everything you missed out on.

Binge eating is sometimes the result of going too long without necessary nutrition and calories. If you consistently skip out on meals when dieting, it is possible to feel deprived and eat many more calories late at night, especially when you're unable to go to sleep from your hunger.

2. Muscle Loss

Unhealthy dieting practices that don't include enough protein can lead to unwanted muscle loss. Your body needs protein to build and repair its tissues, as well as to carry out a large number of body functions and processes. When there isn't enough protein being consumed in your diet, your body will consume its own muscle mass.

3. Fatigue and Nausea

We have talked about the body undergoing those drastic changes and a vast drop in calories and the effects that it has on the body. When you are changing too much at one time, you might feel tried, fatigued and otherwise not well. Some of the most common side effects of unhealthy dieting include dizziness, gate and nausea.

4. Eventual Weight Gain

The challenge with unhealthy diets is that they usually cannot be maintained in the long term. You may be able to survive on an extremely low-calorie diet for short-term, but eventually you will need to resume eating regular meals. When you place yourself on an extreme diet, you don't have the opportunity to gradually develop habits that will help you in the long haul.

It is a much healthier option and you will see greater results in the long term if you adjust your diet gradually. Instead of cutting out thousands of calories on a daily basis, find ways to cut only a few hundred calories each day. Combine those changes with daily exercise.

5. Challenges to Mental Health

Unhealthy dieting is challenging for your mental health on top of the physical problems that it may bring. Many people feel grumpy and irritable when they are hungry and want to eat. Not getting enough calories will leave you not having enough energy to carry out daily tasks, feeling dizzy and nauseous and all of this can all combine together and push some extreme dieters into feelings of deep sadness or sometimes depression.

The best way to avoid these serious consequences of unhealthy dieting is to establish healthy eating patterns. Do this slowly and over time. Identify aspects of your diet that you want to change and work on one change at a time. Reduce your calories gradually. Exercise more than you do. Address your emotional needs. Over time, you will see the pounds fall off and stay off in the long term.

In this book we will look more at weight loss plateaus and help you comprehend what they mean in your exercise regimen. We will also look at easy and practical ways that these plateaus can be minimized or avoided all together and the best success in weight loss can be found. If you are ready to get past all of those weight loss setbacks and finally find the success that you have been looking for, continue reading to get the best information out there.

Why a Plateau with weight loss?

It probably seems very odd to you that this sudden stop in weight change would occur, and it certainly us. But, in the world of medical news and dieting, it is an all too familiar scenario. Your body gets used to what you are doing and eventually it stops trying to defend your body. When this happens, the weight loss stops and it seems that you are stuck between a rock and a hard place without a budget in sight.

There are a few reasons why someone faces the plateau. Yes, it is all related to the weight that you've already lost and the lessened calories that are being consumed, but there are also a few other things that might cause it to happen when you least expect it. You should make yourself aware of all of these things.

More Calories Gone; Lean Body Mass Too?

One of those things is when you take away too many calories. Now, to lose weight it is important that you eliminate some of what you are eating, thus making a reduction in the number of calories that will be consumed on a daily basis. The body needs calories to operate each day even while you are trying to shed the pounds. By doing nothing more than reducing the amount of food that you consume each day, the calories being consumed is also reduced. While your body will still function as it should, it can cause the body to need less calories over time, preventing you from eating the right amount of food to prevent the loss of fat since you are not getting the right calorie intake to restore the lost energy and muscle.

There are a few different ways that you can prevent this from happening to you. One of those is to take things slowly. The body will respond belter when you take things slowly and give it plenty of time to adjust. This means that you should not eliminate more than 500 calories per day off of the menu. When you do not reduce the calorie intake greater than this number you can be sure that your body isn't going to suffer.

Be sure that you calculate the number of calories that you need to consume each day using the basal metabolic rate (or your trusted calculation method.) when you know the number of calories that you need you can easily determine the right amount to take away to keep your body functioning properly.

Another problem that people encounter: they lose lean body mass. As we just talked about it is easy to cause this loss, and it is not something that you want to do. If your metabolism drops, the pounds aren't going to go anywhere, instead clinging to you as good as they can and causing you a lot of frustration.

The Adaption Phase

Once the adaption phase ends, so does the weight loss. Your body responds well to a new exercise regimen or diet plan because it has to make so many different changes to keep up with it. But, your body soon adjusts to the changes and eventually it stops making those adaptions. When this happens, the weight loss also stops. If you want to avoid this, make sure that you are using a variety of exercises in your daily workout, and make sure that high intensity workouts are something that you are participating in. along with having a variety of exercises to perform, you should also change the frequency and the way that you are exercising. When you do this you will prolong the adaption period that your body will go through and phenomenal results can occur.

Are You Doing too Much?

It is very much possible that you are doing too much and the body is stressed out to the max. Over training may be the culprit of the plateau if you are not giving yourself the right method of working out. If you are over training and doing more than what the body can handle, it causes an increase in energy, followed by a big decrease in energy. Make sure that you are exercising regularly, but do not overdo it. If you feel that you are overworking your body, make sure that you give yourself that much needed rest. This is the only way that your body can tell you that you are doing too much, so make sure that you listen to what your body is saying to you. It is okay to rest, to take a break from the norm. As we have already discussed, taking a break and switching things up is the best way to enhance your adaption period and your results. Also remember that you might want to try something different when you resume, and keep things a little but in the light side, at least for a while.

How To Avoid Weight Gain While On Vacation

We look forward to it all year long, but when you're trying to lose weight, vacation could be a damning word. It is while we are relaxing, carefree and with all of our worries left behind while we are on vacation that weight loss can become very difficult. Not only are you aware from home and the surroundings that make you uncomfortable, there's a lot more indulgences around you as well. Fortunately you do not have to miss out on that much anticipated vacation simply because you are trying to lose weight. Take a look at these things that you can do to avoid weight gain while on vacation.

Walk Instead Of Driving

You need a method of transportation while on vacation that is certain. But, whenever possible, walk to your destination. Most hotels are within nearby range of an assortment of activities including dining, entertainment and much more. When you walk you are able to do more exploring while helping you stay on the weight loss train.

Avoid Alcohol

While you may look forward to having a few drinks while on vacation it is best to avoid this task if you are trying to lose weight. Alcohol contains an average of seven calories per gram and also can cause you to overeat. Another downside of drinking is that it can cause you to become inactive.

Eat Sensibly

Vacations can do a number on your diet if you allow it to. Since it is hard to prepare your own meals while you're living it up and staying in a hotel, it is often restaurants that feed our families and us during vacation time. Rather than indulge on the fast food burgers and fries, do as much as you can to stick to your regular eating habits at home. Ask for a healthy menu, and reconsider the restaurants in which you choose to dine at. You can also bring meals with you if they are a part of your weight loss program.

Have Fun

Having fun is what the vacation is all about and sitting back and making sure that you are having fun is a carefree way to ensure that you continue with the weight loss you are trying to achieve. There are a ton of things that you can do while you are on vacation so make sure that you are active and participate in as much as you can for an unforgettable time that doesn't add 10 pounds to your frame before you get back home.

If you are dealing with one of those dreaded plateaus when you do on vacation, do not think that it is a free for all time that you can enjoy anything that you want. This will put all of the progress that you have made thus far back and make you need to work even harder to get where you were at. This is not what you want to happen.

Can a Weight Loss Plateau be avoided?

The weight loss plateau occurs when he body has gotten used to the way that you are doing things. This time period is rarely the same for any two people, but it usually occurs once you have shed about 10 to 11% of your body weight. This is about 5 to 8 months into the regimen for most people, but sometimes it happens before this time, or later for others. There is no way to determine when or if it is something that you will experience so it is best to plan and prepare as if it is going to happen so you can be prepared when it does happen.

If you are like most people, at this point you want to know what can be done to avoid this from happening to you. Sadly, it is not something that you can avoid all together. But, there are numerous ways that you can minimize the risk and the consequences that come along with it. When it is less of a burden you can more quickly resume normal activities and get back to losing weight like you want to lose.

It is kind of obvious that you will see results when you first start working out. The body is enduing something new, and it will try to adapt to that. It is once the body is accustomed to that routine that things become difficult. So, the easiest way to avoid those plateaus s to ensure that you do not keep things routine. Switching things up as we have already talked about will ensure that your body is constantly making adjustments and never settling on the same outline.

Here are some things that you can do to reduce the odds that a weight loss plateau will burden your life.

Make sure that you are watching the portion sizes of the foods that you are eating. We have already talked about this as well, and if you are eating too much, even too much of a good thing, your body isn't going to respond by continued weight loss. Always east smart and according to heart healthy guidelines. There are a number of tools out there that can make it easier to portion out the amount of food that you are consuming per meal. It is a good idea to use one of those tools if at all possible.

Sleep affects us immensely, and oftentimes far greater than what we realize. So, when it comes to sleep and your weight loss you might be surprised to learn that it can have an effect on the outcome. You need to get more than 5 hours of sleep each night, because women who did not were nearly 40% more likely to gain weight. At least 7 hours is recommended, and if you can get 8 or more, good for you. Do not try to sit up 4 days in a row and then make it up for it on the 5th; it won't work and you will likely still feel tired and drained.

Always stay on the move. Even the smallest things really count, so make sure that you are moving around often, even if it is doing nothing but tapping your foot in the floor. If you find a chance to walk instead of drive the car, take advantage of that opportunity. The more active you are the better the results you will find and you will be one step closer to making all of your goals a reality.

How much trans-fat are you consuming? If your diet is high in Tran fat you are far more likely to gain weight. A 5-year research study showed monkeys gained 7% body weight when they had a diet that was high in tans fat.

Before you eat it, wait it out for a period of at least 15 minutes. If you still have the burning desire for that same treat after that time period has elapsed, then indulge if you must.

Find time to relax. Studies have shown that stress can cause a number of problems with the body. It is called the silent killer, after all. If you are stressed it is necessary that the time to relax be taken. Find ways that you can relax and benefit yourself greatly.

Keep in mind that there are also physical factors that affect the plateau that you experience; this can include your age and your gender and the way that your fatty liver and other organs handle the changes. So, just because one-person experiences something one way doesn't necessarily mean that your results will be the same.

Psychological factors can also do a number on an individual who wants to lose weight. There are several things that can cause you to face a hurdle that seems nearly impossible to cross.

Among those factors:

You feel awkward –Sometimes it is hard to be the oddball, especially when you are around friends and other people at social gatherings. But, sometimes it is being the unique person that really draws the attention that you want. Being yourself, being who you really are, will certainly score brownie points with the opal that you want to associate yourself with. There are many ways to bend the rules and still have fun when you are socializing and out with those that you have the most fun.

Comfort Foods: Some people use food to comfort themselves when they feel bad. This is one of the worst habits that you can have because it makes it so much harder to lose the weight. It is essential that you talk to the doctor to learn how to find other means of calming yourself rather than reaching for something to eat.

Low Self-Esteem: Low self-esteem is a big one, and many people who are overweight and carrying around extra weight have these issues. It is hard to get past the low confidence level that you have, but if you can muster through things you are certain to find the rewards very much satisfying in the end.

Depression: Depression is an oftentimes very serious psychological condition that comes with a number of consequences to the person. It can be hard to do normal activities when you are depressed, and suicidal thoughts sometimes occur. Recognizing the signs of depression and getting help for the condition as soon as possible is a must. There are many treatments to help with depression but the first step is seeing the doctor and getting the proper diagnosis. Remember, if you are ever feeling suicidal, call 9-1-1 immediately.

Anxiety: Anxiety can cause stress, panic attacks and more, and there are thousands of people suffering with it every single year. It can also affect the way that you are losing weight and the way that you are able to adhere to the lifestyle changes that comes with your new lifestyle. There are various degrees of anxiety, some of which do require doctor intervention to overcome. So do not be shy if your think anxiety is bothering you.

You Compare Yourself to Others: What one person has is not what is in store for you, so there is no true way to compare yourself to another person on an equal level. You should stop trying to do so. You are your own individual person with your own unique situation and qualities. What is right for one person may not be right for you and you should not want it? Make sure that you live your life for you and do not compare.

Again these are just a handful of the many different psychological conditions that can affect a person. In the most part it is women who are at greater risk for developing one of these conditions, and it is always possible to have more than one or something that is not listed here. If you feel that something just is not right, no matter how minor, get the help that you need.

It is a must that you are able to recognize both the physical and the psychological problems that can affect you and cause trouble when you want to lose weight. It is important to recognize what they are, how they affect you and how to get past them. The first step is simply being able to identify there is a problem and since you are here reading this book, it is apparent that the level you need to be at has been reached and you are ready to go further in your endeavors than ever before.

Overcoming Weight Loss Plateau

What causes your weight to sustain when it reaches a certain point, especially when you haven't changed anything up? There are a number of things that can cause a weight loss plateau. The important thing to remember is that many of these things can be minimized so you are far less likely to suffer. Now, do remember that the plateau is normal, and most people who want to lose weight do experience it. Take a look at some of the common reasons that the plateau occurs.

One of the biggest causes of the plateau is eating too much. You might just be surprised to learn how much you are really eating, and if you are not keeping a journal of these things it can easily get out of hand. It is important that you are always measuring the amount of food that you are consuming as well as the calorie intake. Here are a few pointers that will also help you avoid the pitfalls of the plateau.

Eat a breakfast that is high in fiber. A breakfast of oatmeal is a good idea. When you are eating fiber at breakfast you will feel fuller faster so you will eat less. This important meal gives the brain the fuel that it needs for the day, so make sure that you get it. Another benefit when you eat fiber for breakfast you will to want to eat as much later in the day!

Rather than fill up on sweet or salty snacks when you're hungry or have the munchies, grab a piece of fresh fruit rather than a cookie or other sugary sweet. You will be able to curb your sweet tooth with the fruit while eliminating some of the disadvantages that the sweet treat brings.

When you are adding condiments to your sandwiches or meals, make sure that low-fat versions are chosen whenever possible. You should use the dressings only sparingly, however, as they are often loaded with calories that add drastic numbers to what you are already eating.

Avoid soda. When you are thirsty, water is always your best friend. Sports drinks and green tea are also good choices to aim for. Soda, however, should not be consumed. A cup of coffee each morning is okay, but limit the consumption. Juicing is also very popular these days, and indulging in these very healthy and tasty drinks is something that you can now enjoy at home rather than giving $5 or more for one at the local restaurant.

Use whole grain bread instead of white bread. It is just better for you all the way around.

Learn how to relax and let lose, and always go for the new and unexpected things in life. If you do not it is easy to become bored very fast, and with that boredom it is easy to slip off tack of your weight loss goals. This is certainly not what you want to happen!

Problems when Dining Out

Dining out at a restaurant can be a very tricky situation for someone who is dieting and ready to lose weight. Often times restaurants serve portions far greater than what should be consumed by one persona at any meal, especially for those who are on a diet. In addition it is hard to really know what it is that you are getting. Make sure that you understand you do not have to have an entrée when you dine out. A salad or soup will do if there isn't anything that will accommodate your diet on the menu. You may also want to opt for an appetizer and you can save some money at the same time.

What do You Eat?

You also want to take a look at the foods that you are eating and make sure that you are picking lots of fresh fruits and vegetables. They are high in fiber and low in fat and calories, thus they fill you up and provide you with all of the nutrients that your body needs to thrive. When you are in the plateau, adding more of them to the menu is a really good idea and it will certainly help you get over the hurdle. Make sure that you eat a wide variety of foods, as mentioned before, but when the plateau is on, ensure that it is veggies and fruits that you are pushing.

Push Yourself More

When you are dealing with a difficult time in your weight loss, make sure that you are switching things up a lot. It is variety that helps you succeed and ensures that you are getting the workout that you need. Make sure that you do not stop with simple changes to the exercise however, so make sure that you are pushing yourself more than what you did before. You want to burn more calories and keep the body wondering what is next, so keeping a variety of activities and exercises on the agenda is a good idea.

You can do your regular session with the treadmill, but this time instead of simply walking for half an hour; use a high intensity workout when you start. Also make sure that you switch the routine up with a mixture of strength-training exercises that will help with muscles loss.

You can make small changes such as this every time that you work out. Again, versatility is the key to things; so make sure that you are able to add new workouts with various intensity each day. You can get a nice rotation of things going on and the benefits will certainly be very exciting for you.

Be Patient

Patience is certainly a virtue when you are losing weight. Nothing is going to happen overnight no matter how badly you would like for it to happen. All of those commercials that you see on the TV and the magazine ads of promises telling you that you can shed 20 pounds by next week are nothing more than fads and gimmicks that are doing to cause you more trouble not to mention take your hard earned money for nothing. Do not believe the hype. It is with time, effort and patience that the immaculate results that you want will come your way. You need to eat right, exercise and make other changes that will help you. Make sure that you understand that things do take time and that yon need to wait for it sometimes. This is true of the weight loss plateau as well. Be patient, understand the changes that you need to make, and wait for things to happen smoothly once again.

Listen to Your Body

Your body will never lie to you so make sure that you listen when it gives you a signal that something is wrong. It will always alert you but it is up to you to take the next steps in eliminating the problems.

Weight loss plateaus occur when you are least expecting it, and at what seems the worst possible time for them to occur. Now that you know to expect them to happen, you can better prepare yourself for what is ahead and learn how to deal with it in a more effective manner.

4 Ways To Intensify Your Aerobics Workout

We have mentioned how beneficial it can be to you to add high intensity workouts to your way of doing things, and now we are going to introduce you to a few of the two exercises that you can do to get that intense workout that changes things up and keeps your body in tune and ready to do more.

1. Add an Incline

One of the easiest and most effective ways to make your aerobics routine more intense is to add an incline. Walking, biking, hiking or jogging up an incline will not only make your heart work harder, but it will also engage the muscles in your legs better, resulting in increased muscular strength and tone. When adding an incline to your workout routine, make sure to start out slowly and gradually work your way up. This can be done one or two times per week for phenomenal results. You should try it and see how you like it. It might be a challenge at first but it is certainly something that you can feel good about working toward and accomplished once you are able to retreat the goal.

2. Increase the Speed

Another fun and easy way to make your aerobics routine more intense is to increase the speed at which you're working out. Unlike adding an incline to your workout, which typically limits some of the types of aerobic exercise such as rowing, swimming, or kickboxing, increasing the speed of the activity you are doing is possible no matter what kind of aerobic activity you're doing. Be sure that you increase the speed slowly, and gradually become much faster and faster.

3. Add Variety

In order to really make major changes when it comes to intensifying your current aerobics workout routine, consider varying the types of activity that you're participating in. People often become satisfied with their current fitness routine and perform the same type of activities over and over. This can result in burnout, but can also cause your workout to be ineffective as your body becomes more and more familiar with the exercise. In order to keep your brain and body engaged with what you are doing; make changes to your regular aerobics routine up. For example, one week you can walk or jog, the week you can bike, the following week tries swimming and the last week of the month something else. Continue adding variations to your aerobic routine every month in order to maintain the progress you've been working so hard for.

4. Add Weights

Adding weights to the routine is a great way to make some types of aerobics a bit more challenging. Adding weights to your workout can limit some types of aerobic activity but benefit in many ways. There are many different sizes of weights that you can purchase. If at all possible make sure that you have a variety of weight sizes in pounds so you are always getting a new, fun workout that is intensifying and beneficial to you in every possible way that it can be.

Yoga's Amazing Benefits

Yoga. It has been around for centuries, but has become very popular over the past several years. There are people all around the world who swear by yoga and perform it on a regular basis. They love the benefits, the way that it makes them feel and simply knowing that they are helping their bodies so very much.

Many people wonder if yoga is something that can be used to help a person shed the pounds when they want to lose weight. It seems like yoga would be the perfect source of shedding weight since all of the parts of the body are being worked. But is it really something that you want to try to lose wig doing?

Losing weight with yoga probably isn't something that is going to show significant benefits. But, that doesn't mean that you should not take a look at its awesome benefits that could very well benefit your weight loss endeavors, especially when you are dealing with one of the plateaus that come along.

Yoga can be practiced by men and women of all ages, and with it comes a heightened sense of security, a stronger mind and a stronger body and so much more. Yoga can help an individual relax and gain more confidence, and all of these things are very much needed when dealing with these frustrations of losing weight. When you practice yoga on a regular basis you will become more in tune with your body and can then begin to make better choices for yourself. With that comes more weight loss and less hurdles to overcome to get to the place that you want to be in life.

Although the standard form of yoga may not help you lose weight it can help you to your muscle tone. This is the first of many adventures to come, and a must if you want to lose weight but not your muscles. You will have better posture, so almost instantly you will feel better and regain some of the energy that you have probably lost over time.

There are more intense forms of yoga that an individual can practice if he or she so desires to do so. These do much better at helping an individual lose weight, however, most of them are very hard to perform and take a great amount of skill to master. For this reason most people choose to simply enjoy the awesome benefits that the basic form of yoga offers to them.

Even the basic forms of yoga can be hard to do. It is a good idea that you do not attempt to do them on your own. Make sure that you learn from a certified yoga instructor. There are many different classes that can be found in most any area. The cost of the classes will vary, but you can find an affordable set of classes in a studio near you. Once you learn some of the basics and have gained confidence in completing yoga, taking things home and on a more personalized level may be something that you want to do.

If you have any type of health concerns or health conditions, including problems with the heart or obesity, make sure that you talk to the doctor before you begin this type of regime. There are risks that come along with participating in yoga, and they are a greater risk for those who have health problems already to worry about.

For those who are interested in doing a bit of the high intensity yoga workouts to help them shed a few pounds, there are few types of yoga that are better than the rest. A few of those are:

Power Yoga

Power yoga is what you will likely find being performed at most gyms and is a very popular style of yoga. This form of Yoga uses Astana.

Astana

Astana is one of the most vigorous types of yoga that can be performed. For those who are new to the practice, it is often a series of classes that teaches even the basics. You follow the same group of poses with each workout that you perform when this is the chosen technique of yoga that is followed.

Hot Yoga

Hot yoga is another popular type of high intensity yoga that you might be interested in. it is really fast paced, and well, hot, so you are guaranteed to burn a sweat when you participate!

So, to answer the question of 'will yoga help you lose weight' the answer isn't as simple as what you might like for it to be. Yes, it can help you lose weight, but only if you are doing a lot of it and only if you are doing certain types of yoga. There are far more efficient ways that you can lose weight. But, this isn't to say that you should not use yoga as it provides you with an outstanding number of other benefits that can help you as you attempt to meet all of your weight loss goals. Let's take a final look at the many benefits that yoga can offer to you as you lose weight.

Flexibility: It is no secret that people who participate in yoga are more flexible than the rest of us. Some of the moves that are performed in yoga are quite complex, especially once you begin learning how to do yoga. When you are more flexible, exercising becomes easier and you will find yourself desiring to do more than usual, especially since it is now so much easier to do.

Muscle Tone: You have to tone the muscles if you want a body that is lean and looks great. When you are losing weight, do not forget this important fact, as so many people seem to do. Your body with a lot of weight loss but no muscle tons is not going to be very appealing for you to look at in the mirror, that is for certain.

Relaxation: As mentioned before, stress is not a joke and it is certainly nothing that you want to play around with. It is known as the silent killer, and for a good reason. There are millions of people who die from it each year, or complications of it. If you are stressed out you are doing a grave number on your body and need to begin looking for ways to eliminate that stress. Yoga will help you find that relief. It is great on the body, mind and soul, and with each session you will be able to feel yourself releasing some of the tension that you have inside. Before you know it yoga will be your go-to remedy for stress relief. It works wonderfully, so why not?

Heart Health: Yoga will provide significant results for your cardiovascular health, making it easier to participate in the things that you want to do while also behaving your workout experience. There are far too many people who die from heart attack and heart disease each year, and simple things such as yoga can improve the heart strength and prevent or minima your risks.

Better Sleep: We have already mentioned that you need to get more sleep if you are suffering through a weight loss plateau, and if you are participating in yoga you will certainly be able to get just that. Yoga works almost all of the muscles in the body, and you will feel the burn when you are done. And, since all of those muscles are Bing worked and you are less stressed when you hit the pillows at night it will be for a peaceful snooze for you.

Decreased Risk of Injury: When you are performing yoga you are working your body greatly and improving your flexibility. This does a number of things for you, as we have outlined, including decreasing the risk of injury that you will endure during exercise. It is the muscles that are not accustomed to performing a certain activity that suffer the greatest when exercising. All that it takes is a bit of yoga on a regular basis to minimize those worries. And, with so many other awesome benefits, too, what could go wrong?

Improved Endurance: Another positive attribute with yoga is that you will have an improved endurance. This, too, brings the ability to do more exercise and to have more fun than you ever before.

As you can see, there are some pretty intense benefits that come along with the price of yoga. No matter who you are, these benefits can come your way with the continued use of toga. If you want to enhance your workout, make sure that these are hinges that you are using on a regular basis.

Tips for Weight Loss Success

If you want to lose weight, these are the tips that you need, it is all too often the small things that prevent us from losing weight, however, with these great tips being used you can ensure that you cover all angels of weight loss and achieve the most success.

Tip One: Plan Your Meals

Planning your meals is a great way to ensure that you are testing the things that you need to eat and reducing consumption of those spurs of the moment, most of the time unhealthy food choices. Just as you want to make a shopping list before you head out to the store, you also want to know the meals that you are going to prepare at least one week in advance.

Tip Two: Eat Healthy Fats

Not all fats are bad fats, and you should ensure that you eat foods such as salmon, olives and walnuts, which help you feel more satisfied. They are tasty, too, so that certainly helps things out a lot.

Tip Three: Eat Oatmeal

Oatmeal is an amazing breakfast foods that you should eat regularly. It is rich in fiber as well as grain and it will make you feel fuller so that you're eating less throughout the day. When you want to lose weight this is a must.

Tip Four: Eat Nuts

Along with oatmeal, ensure that you eat a handful of nuts on a regular basis. They'll help you feel fuller. They are a great source of protein as well so when you need to gain a little fuel to make it through the day, those nuts might very well be what you should reach for.

Tip Five: Do not Skip Meals

Skipping meals is a bad idea, as it makes your body go into a fat-storing starvation mode that makes it difficult to burn calories. If you think that this is the way to shed the pounds, think again. You do not want to trick the calories!

Tip Six: Stash a Snack pack

Having an emergency snack pack on hand is a good idea. Your snack pack should contain healthy snack options that will satisfy your craving until it is time for your next meal.

Tip Seven: Shop Smarter

When at the grocery store ensure that you avoid all of those temptations. Make a list before you head to the supermarket and make sure that you make your visits when you're operating on a full tummy.

Tip Eight: Resist Restaurant Temptations

Some restaurants offer appetizers, and you should skip those, as well as any additional extras that are offered, even if they are free. Whenever possible ask the server for a menu of healthy options.

Tip Nine: Slow Things Down

Are you eating too fast? Many people do, and if you are one of those people you could be causing yourself to eat more than what you really want or need to fill you up. Chew your food slowly, and you will enjoy it more while eating less.

Tip Ten: Walk Before You Eat

Before you eat, take a walk. Whether it is a short stroll around the block or a full mile walk, you will eat less when you have added brisk movement to your life. If you would like to see how many steps that you are taking in a single day, a pedometer can be used. These are available in many different locations and are very cheap. These tiny devices keep track of each step that you take throughout the day and they can easily be clipped anywhere on your clothing.

Tip Eleven: Avoid Packaged Snack Foods

Potato chips and similar packaged snack foods may taste great, but they are so bad for you. And, when you use liquid snacks instead you're less likely to overeat. Make sure that you have a nice supply of snacks on hand, including apples, oranges, nuts, rice cakes, etc. These are the stalks that will help you succeed with the weight loss goals that you have in mind.

Tip Twelve: Watch Your Portions

You should ensure portion control is something that you utilize, as the biggest problem with our diets is eating more than what we should. A 9-inch dinner plate should be plenty of room to complete your meal. We have talked about this several times in the book and there is good reason for it. It is so very important for you to keep in mind!

Tip Thirteen: Stay Active

Physical activity is very important. Make sure that you utilize every opportunity that comes your way to get up and move around and stay active.

Tips for Success:

We hope that you have gained a lot of information out of this guide concerning the plateau. We also hope that you have found many different ways to overcome it so that you do not lose out when (and chances are it will come) it happens. The plateau is normal to experience, and while a challenge to overcome, it can be done. The most important thing to remember is to never give up. You can and will succeed if you are not afraid and do not allow the frustrations to overcome you. Handle them with a grain of salt, and make sure that you are ready to fight back and turn out the winner.

In reality avoiding those temptations starts before the actual plateau. There are many things that you can do to help yourself ahead of time and reduce the odds of having problems. As we conclude, we wanted to share with you a few more tips for weight loss success. These tips can be used both before and after your plateau, so make sure that you print this list down, or jot down your favorites, and use them every day as you reach your new self and your new body!

See yourself a Success

When you think you can do something, you can certainly do it. Your mind is very powerful and by simply believing in yourself and putting your mind to doing something, a great victory can be achieved time after time. If you maintain a positive attitude, the chances of being able to lose weight and feel great, even through that difficult plateau stage is more than guaranteed. You are responsible for the future and how things turn out, so if you keep positive, there should be nothing to worry about.

Imagine what you will do once you have shed all of the weight. How great you will look, how amazing you will feel, and even the benefits that it will bring to your health. There are certainly many advantages to being slimmer, including protection against obesity, heart disease and more. Imagine how you will feel when you can get out there and do things with the kids that you have never before, when you can participate in sports and all of the other activities that you were once left out of. You will be able to socialize with friends more, and your positive self-esteem will help you make new friends and meet new people. You'll become more outspoken, Moe individualistic than ever before. Think that you can do it and you will succeed.

Keep A Journal

Words written inside of a journal provide a source of relief and inspiration. You are free to say what you want, to let the pen flow and get it all out there. It is very easy to write those hardships inside of the journal and to express how you really feel without hearing anyone say anything back. You can always go back and look at what you have written to remember a special event or occasion in your life. It is your choice as to how often that you will write in the journal, as well as the topic of content that you will write. It is your space, your paper and your pages to write as you wish, so make sure that you do. Whatever comes to mind, make sure that you put it on paper.

Find a Friend

If you have someone there to support you, it is easier to do almost anything. Whether this is someone that you personally know, someone that you have met on social media or even through an online weight loss forum it is great to be able to talk to this person, to get advice and tips and information when you need it the most. You would be surprised at how much of a difference it can make in your life when you have that needed support. From day one make sure that you have that trusted source there to turn to when times get tough, when you want to talk or simply need someone to push you a little bit harder than before.

Put it All Together

So many people fail to realize that it takes much more than exercise to lose weight. While this is a critical part of success, it is also only one portion of it all. You need to have a well-balanced diet that is filled with a colorful selection of lean meats and fresh fruits and vegetables. You might want to consider eating or sing some of the superfunds that are out there, such as flaxseed, for extra benefits to the health. Remember that all of the exercise in the world will not help you if you're not taking the other measures to lose weight, too. Put it all together and you have an amazing plan!

Eliminate the Temptations

For individuals with families this can get a little tricky, but it is also a great watt to get the whole family in on living a healthier lifestyle. But, it is also a must if you want to find weight loss success. There are many temptations that surround you, and most of them are side of the kitchen pantry and the refrigerator. If you have to stare at these things all of the Tim, eventually you're going to break and indulge. If those temptations are laminated, there is nothing to worry about.

Mistakes Happen

If you make a mistake, it is not the end of the world. Every single day people make mistakes as they try to lose weight because no one is perfect. If this is something that you encounter, do not beat yourself up over it and think that you are doomed from losing weight; you are not. Instead, learn from that mistake and move forward. Every situation that you encounter presents a chance for you to learn from it. No matter what it is or how bad it may seem, you can certainly learn from it if you allow it to happen. Do not think that your diet is over or that all hope is lost because this is far from the situation. We are human beings, and far from perfect. You cannot allow one pitfall to doom you in for life. The most important thing to remember is to recognize your pitfall and make the changes, striving to do better in the future.

Keep a Food Journal

In addition to keeping a journal that you can jot down your thoughts and feelings inside, keeping a food journal is a really good idea. The journal can be used to list all of the foods that you are eating during the day. This can give you a lot of insight to the best methods of shedding those pounds. Your journal can also include menus that you can use each week. Planning your meals ahead of time makes life easier and ensures that you are eating the foods that you need to maintain that good weight and good health. Keep your journal updated, and filled with a variety of foods that you and the family will enjoy.

Make a Shopping List

Before you go to the supermarket, make sure that you have made a shopping list. When you have a list you are less likely to buy those foods that you should not be consuming. It takes just seconds to make the list, and another benefit is that you will also save money when you shop. You should make sure that you have your food journal handy, with the recipes planned for the week, so you know just what you need to buy. But, make sure that you are also getting snacks. Your body craves them, your body needs them, as long as you are making healthier choices and eating sensibly.

Finding A Weight Loss Support Group

Do you want to get that added support of another person to help see you through your weight loss juries? If so there are many weight loss support groups that you should consider. These support groups provide both men and women with a mound of useful advice and information that can greatly benefit them in all of their goals.

Where to Find a Weight Loss Support Group

There are many places that you can find a support group to share your achievements and frustrations with. Oftentimes these support groups are found in obvious places that you simply didn't think to look.

The first place to look for support is the gym where you work out. If there is no message board found in the facility, ask the receptionist if there is a support group around and when and where they meet. The benefit of using a support group found at the gym is that you may also find yourself some friends to work out with along the way.

Another place to look for support is at your workplace. People that work in an office environment can take advantage of this closeness and get together for things like a group walk at lunchtime. Some workplaces even provide an exercise or weight loss program to their employees.

If you participate in any type of group activity, find out if there is a weight loss group. Sometimes church groups and volunteer organizations offer these fitness and weight loss groups.

Finding the Right Weight Loss Support Group

Unfortunately, not all support groups are worthy of your time and fail to encourage positive lifestyle changes and healthy approaches to losing weight. Here are a few tips to avoid such a group.

Is the group competitive? Some of them are, believe it or not. IF this is something that you enjoy, go for it, but it is certainly not right for everyone. These types of groups charge members fees and offer challenges that offer prizes for the winners. If you are up for competition, look into such a group but avoid if you are not.

Make sure that the group that you have chosen to participate in is losing weight in a healthy way. Be cautious of the group if it is dedicated to a fad diet or an unhealthy lifestyle.

If you can't find a weight loss group in your area, do not give up, as there are still a couple of options available to you. Online support groups are available and very popular. You can use them any time of the day or night, and from the privacy of your own home. You can also create your own weight loss group and encourage those around you to be the first members to join.

Many people find that using some sort of tracking system is helpful in ensuring that you are on top of all of your goals. This can help you learn what is beneficial and what is not, enabling you to eliminate things that are not working and focus on what is working instead.

In order to safely lose weight you should take things gradually and combine exercise, healthy eating and determination to do it. It takes weeks to months to shed the pounds in a healthy manner.

Keep an Exercise Log

An exercise log should be kept along with a food journal. Prepare a list of goals for each week of how long you plan to work out, how many exercise sessions you will have and what you'll do for each of those. Keep a close track of the results and enter them in the log, always being honest with yourself. This will help you easily gauge your progress relative to your goals.

Weigh Yourself Regularly

You need to weigh yourself regularly. Choose one day of the week to weigh yourself and do so this day every week, without fail. Record your weight along with the information from your exercise log or your food journal so that you can easily monitor your process. Take a look at the weight difference each week and compare it to the foods that you ate during that period and the exercise that you did the previous week as well.

Weigh Yourself at the Same Time

Your weight fluctuates throughout the day. You may find that your weight loss numbers are somewhat out of order if you are weighing yourself at different times of the day. For this reason, you should always weigh yourself at the same time with every weigh-in. The morning is the best time to weigh yours elf.

Helpful Apps

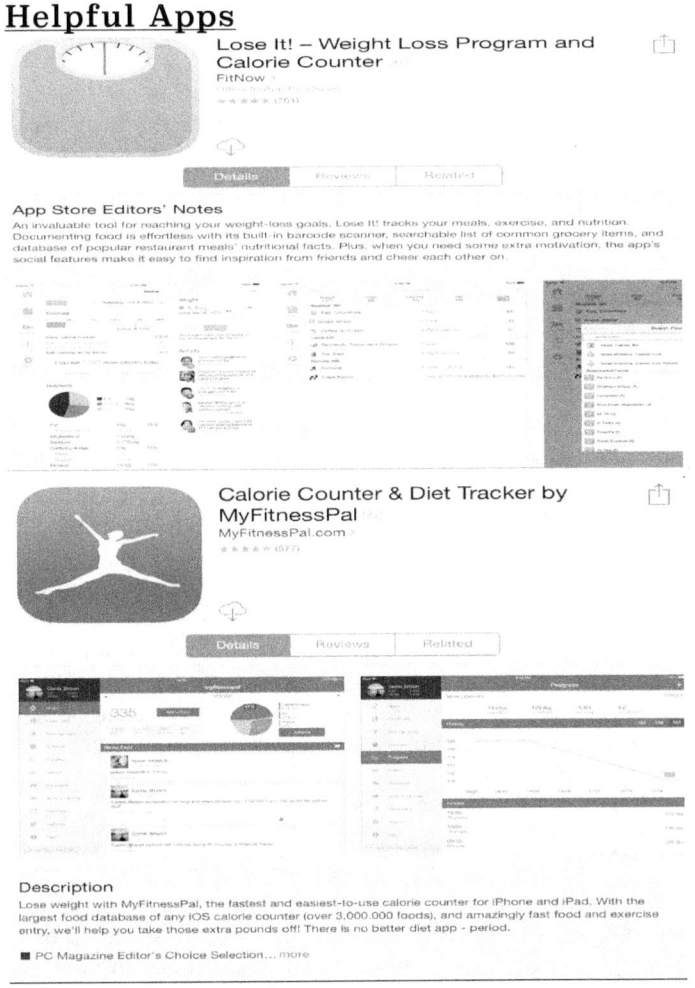

Making Weight Loss Fun

Weight loss success can be yours, and it is a matter of taking the right steps to make losing weight fun. If you think it is not possible to make weight loss fun, think again. Here we offer to you a few tips that can enlighten your workout and show you the fun that it can bring. When you have a fun workout you can have a workout that really provides you with results.

Find an Exercise Partner

It is always better when you have two people. Make sure that you find a friend or family member who wants to get healthy, and together you can head to the gym or plan your workout together. It is much easier to work out when there is someone there to support you, and together you two can provide each other with the utmost of support and motivation. It is certainly a win-win situation for you all.

Reward Yourself

Doing good things for you deserves a reward. When you lose weight, take something unhealthy off of the diet or make another amazing benefit to the program, take the time to give yourself a small reward. You can gift yourself with any gift that you want, whether it is a calorie-free cookie or a trip to the mall for a new item. When you reward yourself you are going to be more inclined to lose more weight and make more changes as there is something there to look forward to.

Enjoy Time with Loved Ones

It is the simple pleasures in life that we must enjoy, even when you want to lose weight. When you are heading outdoors with the kids or the spouse you can do many different activities that will help you lose weight as you enjoy each other's company and something fun to do together. Camping, walking, playing sports, picnics- they're all great ways to get out and benefit your weight loss plans.

Participate in Contests

Weight loss contests can be found far and wide, and oftentimes there are great prizes for those who win. Additionally these contests can help you really focus on your goals of losing weight and help you feel more accomplished at the end of the day. When you're up for a bit of competition and want to enhance the results of your weight loss at the same time, search the web to find such contests and do not hesitate to enter them!

These are just some of the many tips that can help you build the success that you want and need when trying to lose weight. Make sure that you print this list off, or jot them down on paper. They are good for anyone to use, and they can certainly help you. When you are able to combine the tips, the success that is coming your way is enormous.

Good luck and best wishes in your weight loss goals. We know that it is hard, especially when you are on the plateau and want nothing more than to look your best. Nothing is happening and you just do not know what to do about the situation, until now, that is. But, with this information it can be done if you're willing to go the extra mile to make that happen. We hope that you are able to conquer all of the goals that you have in place and get through those plateaus with complete ease. **Anyone can do it, if they put their mind to it.**

About: Dr. A Thomas Spencer

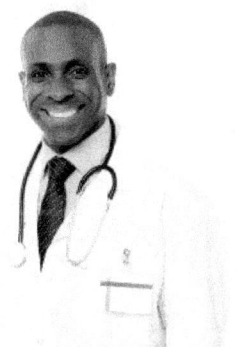

DR. A THOMAS SPENCER is a board-certified family physician that specializes in nutritional researcher and specializes in preventing and reversing disease through nutritional and natural methods.

Growing up with a mother who was a nutritionist, Dr. Spencer learned early on in life about the value of nutrition. He went on to become a success athlete at a prestigious Ivy League school. Once he completed his doctoral studies, he decided to pursue his passion in nutritional research.

He has spent his career as a nutritional researcher and reversing disease through nutrition. "Nutrition is my Life!" a motto that Dr. Spencer conveys to all that know him.

"The quality of our lives can be dramatically altered for the good with great nutrition habits. You are what you eat means something. Nutrition is one of the most important facets in our lives. We must build great habits everyday. Those habits can be passed from generation to generation. You are only given one body in your lifetime. Feed that body with premium nutrition. Always remember that racecars do use 87-octane fuel. Why shouldn't you?"

-DR. A.THOMAS SPENCER

Finally, if you enjoyed this book, please take the time to share your thoughts and post a review on Amazon. It'd be greatly appreciated!

How To Lose Belly Fat Fast

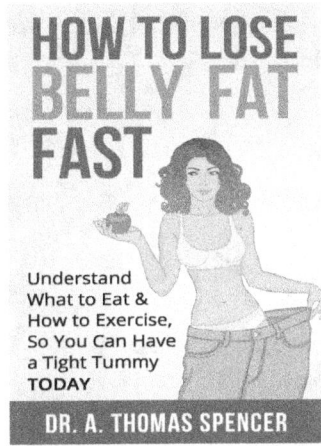

THE BEGINNING OF A NEW YOU:

We have a layer of fat under the skin called subcutaneous fat. This fat makes up about 80-90% of our total body fat and is typically located on the back of the arms, below the shoulder blades, around the belly and on the upper legs and hips. The remaining 10-20% of our body fat is termed belly fat, also known as visceral fat, and is located beneath the stomach muscles and around internal organs such as the liver, spleen, intestines and kidneys. In some people, belly fat can also accumulate in organs such as the liver. Interestingly, people who have more fat on their upper thighs have less incidence of type 2 diabetes and cardiovascular disease. Subcutaneous fat serves a number of purposes, such as keeping us warm and acting as a storage site for hormones and energy. Also called adipose tissue, it used to be thought of mainly as a ready source of energy in times of famine, but fat is now viewed as an endocrine organ that stores and excretes a number of hormones and chemicals that can have both positive and negative effects on health. Fat mass secretes over 30 chemical messengers, some messengers, such as the hormone leptin, tell the brain that we have had enough to eat, whereas other chemicals, such as tumor necrosis factor, a cytokine, and induce inflammation to help to combat pathogens.

Belly fat accumulation is influenced by a number of factors, such as possessing high levels of fat storing hormones and low levels of fat burning hormones, being sedentary and having certain genes. Eating too much processed food is also related to belly fat accumulation include age, ethnicity and lifestyle.

Unique Causes of Belly Fat:

Fat storing hormones:

Cortisol, a hormone that is secreted into the blood by the adrenal glands, is typically elevated when people experience stress. When blood cortisol levels increase, the amount of sugar in the blood also increases, which results in a corresponding rise in insulin. Having elevated levels of cortisol and insulin in the blood encourages fat storage and impedes fat burning. This means high levels of stress increase the levels of cortisol and insulin in your blood, leading to reduced fat release and increased belly fat stores. Cortisol may also contribute to leptin resistance, which means people eat more, as leptin is a satiety hormone that fat cells release to tell the brain we have had enough to eat.

Fat burning hormones:

In humans, catecholamines are the major hormones that mobilize fat from fat cells and induce fat burning in muscles and the liver. The catecholamines are epinephirine and norepinpehrine and are secreted into the blood by the adrenal glands. Norepinephrine is also released at nerve endings. Blood catecholamine levels gradually increase through the night and typically peak around 11am. Catecholamine induced fat mobilisation occurs much more in belly fat compared to subcutaneous fat.

Another fat burning hormone is growth hormone, which is produced by the pituitary gland. Insulin slows down growth hormone release, so people with high levels of insulin in their blood typically have lower levels of growth hormone. Having problems with the thyroid gland can also result in increased belly fat accumulation. The thyroid is an endocrine gland located at the base of the neck and release a hormone called thyroid hormone, which elevates metabolic rate and, together with catecholamines and growth hormone, increases fat release from cells. Hypothyroidism occurs when the thyroid gland produces too little thyroid receptors in cells become insensitive. Low thyroid levels can contribute to elevated fat deposition and can cause an increase in belly fat stores and are often accompanied by elevated low-grade inflammation, as hypothyroid individuals have been shown to possess increased levels of C-reactive protein, an inflammatory chemical, in their blood.

Genetic influences:

Over the last 3 decades, researchers have discovered genetic markers that contribute to increased body weight and waist circumference, however no single gene has been found to cause obesity. Specific genes related to obesity have been identified among them are a number of single gene mutations that contribute to the development of obesity in teenagers and young adults. This means we now know that genes affect belly fat development when influenced by factors such as physical inactivity, nutrient intake and metabolic status.

Lifestyle factors that influence belly fat cause:

There are many lifestyle factors that impact on belly fat, but perhaps the most important are age, drinking alcohol, ethnicity, smoking, stress and sleep. Exposure to daily stressors and reduced quality of sleep has both been associated with belly fat accumulation.

Physical inactivity:

People who do not do recreational exercise and have little physical activity in their jobs are prone to belly fat accumulation, especially if they consume a lot of processed food. This belly fat accumulation risks developing cardiovascular disease, as well as type 2 diabetes. Exercising burns up energy and gradually makes the body metabolize more fat than carbohydrate. It is also likely that fat burning continues during the period after exercise.

Age:

Older people tend to have more belly fat than young people. The main reason for the increase in belly fat in older people seems to be a decrease in the body's metabolism, after the age of 30, most people's metabolism will decrease about 1% every 2 years. Why metabolism slows as we age is unclear, but it probably involves a decrease in muscle mass and a change in hormone levels. While the amount of subcutaneous fat generally declines with ageing, so does muscle mass, and since skeletal muscles, together with the liver, are the major fat burning engines of the body, older people burn lower levels of fat overall.

Alcohol:

Alcohol contains 7 calories per gram, which is more than 5 calories contained in a gram of carbohydrate and protein, and just under the 9 calories per gram contained in fat. Thus, consuming 2-3 average sized alcoholic drinks a day adds up to over 500 calories. In a week, over 3500 extra calories would be consumed. Since 1 calorie equals 9 grams of fat that means having 3 drinks every day of the week add almost 400g of fat to your diet. According to studies in this area, the majority of these calories appear to be deposited as belly fat. It has also been shown that consuming alcohol makes people hungry.

Smoking:

Typically, smokers weigh less than non-smokers as, smoking may reduce appetite and also elevate metabolic rate, which induces fat burning. There is evidence, however to show that cigarette smoking increase belly fat accumulation a large population based study in the UK found that men and women who smoked possessed increased belly fat. How smoking increases belly fat is unclear, but shortly after a smoker finishes a cigarette, blood cortisol levels can increase for up to 30 minutes. We know that cortisol can increase belly fat accumulation due to its effect on blood sugar and insulin levels. Smokers also exercise far less than non-smokers, which is also likely to contribute to increased belly fat accumulation.

How to Lose Belly Fat Fast:

Getting started on a diet:

Prior to starting on a diet, you need to make sure that you are fully committed about it. In other words, you need to have the discipline and the determination to follow through it, in order to attain your fitness goals. Aside from that, you should also have the right motivation to stay on track.

What Burns calories?

Calorie Burning Chart				
Activity	150 lbs.	165 lbs.	180 lbs.	195 lbs.
Aerobic Dance	170	187	204	221
Calisthenics	119	131	143	155
Cycling (5.5 mph)	136	150	163	177
Dancing	102	112	122	133
Golf (with cart)	119	131	143	155
Housework	102	112	122	133
Hiking – cross country	204	225	245	265
Jump Rope (slow)	272	299	327	354
Racquetball	238	262	286	310
Rollerblading	374	412	449	486
Running/jogging	238	262	286	310
Skiing – downhill	204	225	245	265
Skiing – cross country	272	299	327	354
Sitting – office work	51	56	61	66
Stair climbing	272	299	327	354
Stretching	85	94	102	111
Swimming	238	262	286	310
Tai Chi	136	150	163	177
Walking (3 mph)	112	123	135	146
Walking, brisk (4 mph)	129	142	155	168
Weight training	102	112	122	133
Yard Work – gardening	136	150	163	177
Softball	170	187	204	221
Squash	408	449	490	531

www.ingramcontent.com/pod-product-compliance
Lightning Source LLC
Chambersburg PA
CBHW060154290526
45789CB00003B/1040